T0342442

THE RISE OF MENTAL VULNERABILITY AT WORK

A Socio-Historical and Cultural Analysis

Ari Väänänen

First published in Great Britain in 2024 by

Policy Press, an imprint of
Bristol University Press
University of Bristol
1–9 Old Park Hill
Bristol
BS2 8BB
UK
t: +44 (0)117 374 6645
e: bup-info@bristol.ac.uk

Details of international sales and distribution partners are available at
policy.bristoluniversitypress.co.uk

British Library Cataloguing in Publication Data
A catalogue record for this book is available from the British Library

ISBN 978-1-4473-5942-5 hardcover
ISBN 978-1-4473-5943-2 paperback
ISBN 978-1-4473-5944-9 ePub
ISBN 978-1-4473-5945-6 ePdf

Cover design: Nicky Borowiec
Front cover image: Adobe Stock/dbrus
Bristol University Press and Policy Press use environmentally responsible print partners.
Printed and bound in Great Britain by CPI Group (UK) Ltd, Croydon, CR0 4YY

FSC
www.fsc.org
MIX
Paper | Supporting
responsible forestry
FSC® C013604

Contents

Acknowledgements

Several highly skilled colleagues have collaborated in this long-term project. I would particularly like to mention Erkko Anttila, Anna Kuokkanen and Pekka Varje, who have offered their thoughts, ideas, counterarguments and hard work that have pushed this project forwards. Over the past years, research work with Pauliina Mattila-Holappa and Kristiina Lehmuskoski has provided me numerous fruitful discussions and opportunities to understand our research target in a new way. There have also been numerous other colleagues and researchers in Finland and abroad who have helped myself and my team in this task. Especially, Iain Wilkinson and Tim Newton have provided me an opportunity to discuss the subject area over the years, offering highly needed support and generously sharing their views and ideas. The insightful comments made by Vilma Hänninen and Juha Sandberg were very helpful in the process of clarifying several parts of the manuscript. The luxury of having support from Elisa Falck, Emma-Reeta Käsmä and Rosa Aphalo provided me with a chance to elaborate my text and contributed to the preparation of this book in several ways. I would also like to mention Jorge Belmonte from the University of Valencia, which whom I discussed the preliminary thoughts on this topic in the early 2000s. Those chats led to critical studies on work stress and occupational health, which have been one of my key research areas, intimately associated with the topic of the societal emergence of mental vulnerability. At the end, I would like to mention my colleague and friend Jussi Turtiainen with whom I have had joyful and stimulating collaboration over many years while trying to solve the puzzle of mental vulnerability of our age. Without Jussi this book would have looked quite different. In addition, the person who has significantly influenced the content and presentation of the themes of my research work with her sharp arguments and sparring is my spouse and colleague Minna Toivanen. I would like to express my deep gratitude to all of you as well as many unnamed others who have contributed to the birth of this text.

This work has been funded by the Finnish Cultural Foundation, the Research Council of Finland (#345170, project LIFECON), the Association of Finnish Nonfiction Writers and the Committee for Public Information. Its realization has also been facilitated by a wide range of support from the Finnish Institute of Occupational Health across the years. I would like to thank all these parties for making the book possible.

Preface

I will start the story with my father. He was born in a sauna (a common custom in Finland at that time) in a small village in Eastern Finland close to the Russian border in the first spring of the 1930s. Because of the war, he had a fragmented schooling which only lasted a few years. As he grew up, he started to work at the family farm in the 1950s. Due to musculoskeletal problems, diminishing possibilities for a decent living in the remote countryside of Finland and growing urban labour markets he decided to sell his farm in the 1960s and started a new job as a district inspector in an insurance company in the largest town of Eastern Finland, Kuopio, in 1966. In Kuopio, he met my mother, who had also moved from the countryside to the city some years earlier. They met when my father came to sell an insurance policy to my mother.

While I was a child in Kuopio in the 1970s, most of my friends had a similar family background. Their parents had grown up in the countryside, had moved to the town, and most of them had started to work in services, healthcare or sales. Most of them did not have long-term academic education. At weekends and on holidays, we often travelled to the countryside where our relatives still lived. In the countryside, the livelihood was based on agriculture and cattle-raising. People woke up early in the morning to take care of the animals and many food supplies came from their own land. Many jobs depended on the weather and the changing seasons. The language and the customs were also different: in the countryside the dialect was stronger, and the role of religion was more important than in the city. Contemporary social scientists of the 1960s and 1970s interpreted the era of my childhood as a period of 'structural transition' which was often marked by a rapid change in the occupational structure, urbanization, the birth of suburbs, rapid material improvements and changes in the mode of life (Haapala, 2004).

In the 1980s, Finland became one of the wealthiest countries globally and schools, hospitals and different services reached the standards of a rich welfare country. The younger generation got used to a world that looked much more urban and international than the world of their parents. In our lives, chain cinemas, pizzerias and cheap French and German wines became the new normal. We sat in cafés and spent our time driving in circles around the city and listening to rock music on cassette tapes. MTV provided us with up-to-date information on the international music scene. We played tennis on summer evenings and ice hockey in winter. My friends and I graduated from high school in 1987 and went Interrailing in the summer, seeing ten countries in a month. We wanted to disengage ourselves from the circles of a small town and had a heart-aching desire to see Europe. Soon everything changed. Many of us left our hometown in the late 1980s as we started to study or work in the bigger cities of Southern Finland. The speed of economic growth gave us confidence regarding the future.

I initiated my studies in social psychology at the University of Tampere two months before the Berlin Wall fell in 1989. Our department was strongly impacted by the critical social psychological tradition influenced by American interactionism, Russian psychology and Anglo-American critical strands. Positivism and standard methods of social research and mainstream psychology were heavily criticized. I visited my hometown, parents and relatives every now and then, but daily life was centred around academic circles and new friendships.

I completed my studies in social psychology in 1997 and started my final period of psychological practice in April 1998 at the Finnish Institute of Occupational Health in Helsinki. I was supposed to learn practical skills necessary for a practising psychologist, but reality offered me a different path as I was located to a research unit which was studying job burnout, sickness absence and other occupational health issues from a psychosocial perspective. I had training and a background as a critically oriented social scientist and psychologist and as a critical psychologist but suddenly I found myself in the world of work psychology characterized by research on job characteristics, personality types and symptom scales. Suddenly I was in the area of mainstream applied psychology and quantitative methods, with which I was not familiar.

I stayed at the Finnish Institute of Occupational Health and became a researcher. Gradually I learnt new concepts and theoretical models and became familiar with statistical techniques and software. I became acquainted with scientific writing skills and started to prepare manuscripts to be submitted to international journals. I worked with several excellent researchers from Finland and other countries. However, while investigating I repeatedly found myself considering why we used these concepts, these models and these understandings. Why psychosocial factors and stress explanations? Why causal pathways and mediations? Or more analytically: Why do these discursive frameworks rise? How do these ways of seeing and conceptualizing our labour market and occupational health dampen the influence of human behaviour and culture as they remain focused on mechanisms and variables? I ended up questioning how we as scientists try to capture the problems of psycho-emotional functioning and challenges at work.

Gradually I started to look for something that could explain the emergence of these topics, ideas, models and arguments. Individual-level measurements and modelling became less important while employees and professionals operating in their culture and parsing issues of work and wellbeing became the focus of my research. I started to investigate historical and cultural tendencies that possibly gave birth to approaches representing and measuring 'burnout-subjects', 'psychosocial resources', 'stress factors' and 'coping strategies'.

Looking back, I see numerous circumstances, coincidences and contradictions in my autobiographical past, that have produced the need to write about this subject. Using these pieces, in hindsight, I can develop a narrative that describes why I ended up writing this book. I may even state that there are several issues in my personal history that have impacted the content of this book, such as my childhood experiences, distancing myself from my parents, and the scientific and ideological conflict of distinctive traditions taking place in my own life as a researcher. The list could be much lengthier.

Personal life events, circumstances and emotions are unique to me. They have developed in my social contacts and personal experiences along my life course. However, the individual experience I feel meaningful to narrate is embedded in the broader social, economic and cultural history. My agency, my problems, my worldviews, and even my inner motivations could not be possible without the history of this Northern European country, its rapid development and the contradictions caused by this. At the same time, wider European and even non-European history is filtered through my society and social relationships. My thoughts and emotions regarding occupational health, mental health at work and psychology are emerging as I write in a small room but relate to numerous others in the past and present.

In this book, I will try to understand the history- and culture-bound social behaviour of employees and professionals. In the discourses of work and health dominated by wellness consultants, mental health specialists and organizational developers this book intends to offer an alternative counter-storyline. From the context of critical social theory, it tries to offer a more grassroots level perspective on the history of occupational health, mental health and work culture than most critical books on work stress, work-related health or governing of employees in late modern societies. As the point is to focus on 'history in the making', it is important to listen, document and analyse the products and arguments of the history makers.

The rapid modernization that took place in Finland from the 1950s to the 2000s offers a particular window for this historically orientated macro-social psychological study. From this perspective, it was not unique that my father happened to be a farmer in the 1950s and moved to the capital of the geographic area in the 1960s, while I happened to become a knowledge worker in the late 1900s. In the Finland of the 1960s, three-quarters of the farmers' sons, and even a larger proportion of their daughters, left their parents' occupation (Haapala, 2004: 253), while in the early 2000s about one-quarter of the population were knowledge workers in Finland (Väänänen et al, 2016). Due to such drastic structural transitions in the forms of living and working, it can be argued that Finnish working-age generations and occupational health professionals of the past decades have been operating in the context of a 'compressed' experience of modernization (Beck and Grande, 2010). For this reason, in my studies with my colleagues, I have assumed that by focusing attention on transformations within the working knowledge, experience and narrations of Finnish employees, media and other 'socio-cultural producers' between 1950 and 2020, we are provided with a unique opportunity to study the changing arena of mental health.

This book explores how mental-health-related social opportunities and frameworks were gradually built under transforming cultural and occupational circumstances. It also describes how psychological knowledge, professional interventions and scientific approaches started to be called for in the regulation of emotional life among employees. It elaborates an analysis of the transition of the mental landscape that produced new arenas recognizing subjective experiences and a phenomenon that is commonly understood as a mental health crisis. Although my focus is on mental health and problems of mental coping related to work capacity, my analytical focus is not on the individual level. I merely study how people living in a certain historical period and circumstances (both lay and professional) signal, reconstruct and share ideals, norms and moralities that are related to the social and organizational life and how they understand the status of the psyche and describe it. I also study the problems they describe and bring up at work and look at how they have changed over a long period of time. In this way, this book attempts to develop a new way of understanding the emergence of the mentally troubled subjectivity and its initial roots in our history.

Friedrich Nietzsche pointed out how it is important to study the history of self-evident truths and analyse how power is involved in truthmaking while the Annales school of French historians has stressed the importance of studying long-term historical periods in the formation of ways of thinking, 'mentalities'. In turn, Norbert Elias has described how behavioural codes and strategies among people have changed during the centuries and self-regulation in the processes of 'civilization'. French social theorist and historian Michel Foucault has formulated many ideas of how we are gently governed and attached to various 'normalizing practices' as citizens and professionals. These models of thought have encouraged me to think that it is possible to study social codes of emotional behaviour, standards of work capacity, nature of identity demands, and other historical characteristics involved in crafting mental vulnerability as a part of the late modern self and work.

Background: mental health crisis in the labour market

Mental health crisis of late modernity

Over the past decades, one of the most striking health-related trends in Western working-age populations has been the growth of challenges and concerns related to mental health. International institutions (for example, the World Health Organization [WHO], European Union [EU]) and national governments have repeatedly raised the crisis of mental health and increasing burden of mental disabilities as priorities on their agendas while economists have estimated the immense burden to national economies as billions of work years are lost and the efficiency of work is weakened due to poor mental health (Trautmann et al, 2016). If we take mental health statistics as the objective compass of information on mental health, we observe dramatic trends across developed societies. In the United States and Europe, the number of people treated for depression multiplied between the late 1980s and early 2000s (Mojtabai, 2008; Marcus et al, 2010) and the proportion of anxiety-related health problems began to rise at an unexpected rate (McDaid, 2008; Schnittker, 2021).

Today mental health is no longer a side issue in the well-off societies in terms of the population's vitality. In the countries belonging to the Organisation for Economic Co-operation and Development (OECD, 2015), mental disorders account for 30–50 per cent of all long-term sickness and disability in the working-age population. In many EU countries, more than half of disability pensions and benefits are related to mental problems (Nyman and Kiviniemi, 2015; Viola and Moncrieff, 2016), and mental disorders are one of the largest contributors to chronic conditions (years lived with disability) affecting the population of Europe and the United States (Ferrari et al, 2022). The WHO has ranked depression (2017) as the single largest contributor to global disability (7.5 per cent of all years lived with a disability in 2015). For instance, in 2018–2019 depression or anxiety were responsible for 44 per cent of all cases of work-related ill-health and 54 per cent of all working days lost due to health issues in Great Britain (Health and Safety Executive, 2019). The growth of mental-health-related problems and disabilities has also been pronounced in high-income welfare countries such as Canada and the Nordic countries, especially among young adults (Sommer, 2016; Côté, 2019; Madsen, 2021). Faced with drastic change, some social scientists have suggested that the challenge of mental health is one of the key crises of late modernity (for example, Rosa, 2019).

A noticeable rise in work disability due to mental disorders has also been found in recent years in Finland, which is an empirical 'case country' of this book. This has now become a priority on the Finnish public health agenda, particularly concerning young age groups and disability retirement (Sumanen et al, 2016; Hakulinen et al, 2019). In 2021, 36 per cent of all compensated sickness absence days were due to mental disorders. Among those aged 20–29, mental disorders contributed to 64 per cent of all compensated sickness absence days in 2021. Of all disability pensions in Finland, 33 per cent were granted due to mental disorders. Among those aged under 35 years, 83 per cent of disability pensions were granted due to mental disorders (Finnish Centre for Pensions, 2022; Social Security Institution of Finland, 2022a).

At the same time, the difficulties attached to mental health such as depression and anxiety have raised public concern both in various branches of science and on numerous media forums. Not only problems categorized as mental disorders but also numerous associated problems such as work stress, exhaustion and psychological distress have become major societal issues and common concerns (Väänänen et al, 2014; Schaufeli, 2017). On the face of it, this has been unexpected. Why do current generations born in welfare societies seem to have far more problems with their psyche than earlier generations? We may also ask how our narratives, definitions and subjective experiences have been occupied by a variety of mentally taxing emotions and why these 'problems of the mental' are increasingly understood as key reasons for not being able to work. In this book, using various materials and scientific discussions, I aim to find how this change has occurred both in work and in the behaviour of the working-aged. To understand the challenged psyche of the working-age population I shall dig into the roots of mental health centrality and the emerged problem of challenged mental ability in the workforce using historical, interview, register and theoretical materials from a variety of scientific disciplines.

The growing concern on mental fitness

To understand the current emergency with mental health among working-age people there is a need to look back and see how these 'epidemics' started to emerge and what we had before them. Already in the 1950s, but especially in the 1960s some American and European researchers and labour market reformers (for example, Kornhauser, 1962; Herzberg, 1968; Thorsrud, 1970; Gardell, 1976) were worried about the monotonous nature of industrial work and they observed that certain forms of exhaustion and fatigue were not solely caused by physical strain but rather related to psychological, social and emotional features of work. In the early 1970s, more public attention on mental health problems was received in other types of occupations as well when job burnout symptoms emerged as a serious problem among healthcare workers in the United States (for example, Freudenberger, 1974). Scholars of the new generation began to explore how 'psychosocial' aspects could affect employees' mental health (for example, Kornhauser and Reid, 1965; Katz and Kahn, 1966; Frankenhaeuser and Gardell, 1976; Emery and Thorsrud, 2013 [1969]). At this time, especially work stress was recognized as a source of poor mental wellbeing, which led to the development of the new occupational health models and theories on the psychobiological crafting of mental distress in industrial and organizational psychology as well as occupational health research in general (for example, Cooper and Marshall, 1978; Levi, 1978; Warr, 1987, 2007).

During the 1980s, the research on the psychological outcomes of industrial work began to expand into white-collar occupations, which had started to dominate the map of occupational structure in Western countries (Väänänen et al, 2012). In the management organizations, and among experts, much more attention towards work stress, burnout and psychological overstrain started to disseminate. Older workers, public sector workers, temporary workers, knowledge workers, workers in female-dominated occupations, and various other groups moved to a risk zone where their psychological and emotional resources were threatened.

By the beginning of the new millennium, numerous concepts entered the stage that described the lack of psychic energy and problems of mental distress among employees. This was seen quantitatively in the growth in the amount of studies on burnout, depression and stress (Wainwright and Calnan, 2002, 2011; Friberg, 2009; Väänänen et al, 2014). Although national differences were present at the conceptual level, post-industrial societies had reached a consensus related to endangered public health and work ability due to poor mental health among the workforce and/or potential workforce. Although the interest in adequate functioning of citizens and population vitality grew considerably in the 19th century in many leading Western national states moving towards modernity (for example, Greenfeld, 1992), the humanitarian enterprise of the late 20th and early 21st century aiming at the mental capacity of the workforce had a far more psychological and mental health-focused character. The psychological vitality of the active population who were supposed to be productive and able to support citizens unable to work was at stake. In 2009, based on the research of a considerable number of established public and occupational health researchers, the director of the European Agency for Safety and Health at Work concluded:

> Work-related stress is one of the biggest health and safety challenges that we face in Europe. Stress is the second most frequently reported work-related health problem, affecting 22% of workers from the EU

27 (in 2005), and the number of people suffering from stress-related conditions caused or made worse by work is likely to increase. (Takala, 2009: 7)

At the same time, historically unforeseen physical health has developed and flourished in many countries that are occupied by mental health concerns. For instance, life expectancy was at a record high level on a global scale in most EU countries in the early 21st century (Knudsen et al, 2019). Material wealth has improved with immense speed and the prevalence of traditional health problems such as cardiovascular diseases has declined considerably since the 1970s (Kouvonen et al, 2014; Bhatnagar et al, 2016). In addition, several improvements have been seen in terms of a decline in occupational diseases (occupational asthma, hearing loss, musculoskeletal problems) and fatal injuries (Hämäläinen et al, 2009; Stocks et al, 2015) in most European countries. It appears that material affluence and physical health have not created mental fitness and psychological wellness among working-age adults.

The mental health crisis becomes an even more intriguing puzzle if we note that especially since the 1990s there has been a strong and fast-growing research and consultancy field stressing the role of positive wellbeing and resource-based thinking in the context of work. One of the main observations in positive work and mental health psychology has been that a vast majority of mental health outcomes both in psychology as well as psychiatry have been based on symptom and disorder-driven thinking and modelling, thus risk factors and negative outcomes instead of positive emotions and wellbeing (Seligman, 2002; Turner et al, 2002; Bakker and Schaufeli, 2008). As the positive perspective has gained ground in both the sciences and the consulting field, is it reasonable to ask, why it does not seem to help the psychological ill-feeling of the working-age population. Is this the dominance of psychiatric discourses stressing disorder-based thinking, diagnostics and old-fashioned psychology emphasizing negative illnesses instead of positive wellbeing? Or do we have such high demands and obligations in the cognitively and socially fully loaded economy that the interventions of behavioural sciences focused on grassroots-level changes cannot resolve it? Is it even justified to expect that any discipline or perspective could capture this multifaceted challenge in a satisfactory way?

The need for rethinking mental health in the context of work

When I write about mental health in this book, I am not parsing it from the framework of individual health but as part of the changing understanding, definition and management efforts of employees' social and emotional behaviour and its challenges. I treat mental health as a phenomenon whose cultural expansion I analyse. Because of this perspective, the aim of the book is not to seek better mental health, but rather to produce information about the essential processes that have put mental health on a pedestal and made it an essential way of looking at work and the working-age population. Thus, when I write about the expansion or spread of mental health, I do not mean the improvement of the mental health of the population, but the growth of the area and cultural role of mental health.

I will particularly aim to raise and analyse the key production- and culture-related mechanisms between the 1960s and the early 2020s that have provoked the emergence of the great mental health invasion entangled with each other. Because the phenomenon is closely related to changes in occupations, expert knowledge and cultural codes of behaviour, I aim to base my arguments and observations on interview and archival sources collected over a long period of time and amplify the analysis using scientific literature I see as fruitful in terms of developing the analysis. This approach may be criticized for being too eclectic in terms of scientific research, but as my main intention is to shed light on the historicity and social nature of mental health, work ability and occupational health in general, I will prioritize this content-driven aim and try to keep all necessary parts in my analysis.

There are numerous scientific areas that could be useful in the study of a society and work which are susceptible to mental problems, but these areas have largely remained separate. However, perspectives developed by work scholars, social historians, social theorists, epidemiologists, critical and work psychologists, organizational researchers, cultural anthropologists, and many other scientific scholars can jointly bring new perspectives to the area of mental health and work.

In research on mental health and work, I have been worried about four interrelated issues. First, the main body of research on work–related mental health in our society mainly lacks a historical socio-cultural perspective. This makes us blind to whether these issues are unique to our time and how these concerns may have developed during history and go beyond our own daily existence. Maybe we had mental health problems before we understood that this was a mental health crisis that should be dealt with. Second, the analyses of mental health have been dominated by individualistic approaches and methodologies. We have been accustomed to viewing mental health as something that is produced by individual trajectories such as poor childhood conditions, traumatic events, genetic makeup, risk factors of the working environment and so on. This perspective of individualism limits our understanding of immediate risk factors and relegates the transition of culture and work to the footnotes. However, without understanding the fundamental transitions in occupational life and society transforming mental health and its cultural status, it is very unlikely to reach a proper understanding of the emergence of the mental health crisis in post-industrial societies.

Third, there are various sophisticated analyses of the emergence of cultural processes (for example, individualization), labour market changes (for example, neoliberal economy) and other unequalizing processes, and how they have been reflected in psychological distress among working-age people. These analyses have provided valuable insights into the origins of the mental health invasion. However, they are often bound in different theoretical perspectives and there is a lack of interaction between them. There are surprisingly few analyses of how our historical agency at work has changed and how different generations have crafted social worlds, what kind of burdening experiences they have had in their daily life and how they have seen the role of emotional management in their lives. Fourth, the concept of mental health is understood as a part of mental states and mechanisms of the individual mind. In the media, as well as expert debates, this view on human mental health offers us the cognitive framework under which mental health is discussed. The dominance of health perspective directs us to think about the individual's health. When the perspective is broadened beyond the different historical periods and cultures, a new question arises: To what extent is the issue in the area of health? Could the whole phenomenon be better understood by looking at what possibly makes large population groups turn towards mental health?

Health sociology has suggested that, in Western post-industrial societies, health in general has come to depend less on the biological and physical environment and much more on social, cultural and behavioural factors (for example, Petersen and Wilkinson, 2008). But what are these 'environments' and 'factors'? I would also continue to ask whether this really is a mental health crisis or whether we are dealing with something else. I argue that we would need to dig into the social arenas of employees and society that made psychological worries and distress a part of our subjectivity and its challenges. Instead of asking what is wrong in our work environment or with our personal relationships or personal past, should we instead ask questions such as: What propels the engines of vulnerability and what are its benefits? How is our behaviour at work characterized by knowledge about mental vulnerability? Why is mental health needed today in our current social existence and why did past generations not need it as we do?

In this sense, this book has a certain ontological and epistemological basis. I am concerned with how we 'understand' mental health, work ability/disability and risks related to occupational life, 'what they are' and 'how we know what they are'. Even though this sounds like philosophy of science, each research project and development programme dealing with mental health and wellbeing among working-age individuals is guided by a set of assumptions, whether it is the classic positivist assumption that occupational health and mental health as its subsection can be straightforwardly known through 'reliable' and 'valid' measurements, or the 'strict' constructionist position that maintains that all representations of organizational life and work-related mental health are necessarily fallible and subject to ongoing contestation and dispute (Newton et al, 2011). All in all, we need to rethink the fundamental assumptions and interrelationships concerning psyche, emotions, work, health and work ability in current society, and how we began to understand mental health issues as we know them today.

If we compare the situation of the early 2020s with the situation in the 1970s, the transition has been tremendous. Perspectives, classifications, measurements, samples, concepts, institutional arrangements and needs for care have experienced an accelerated change. Even though research on work generally look at the big changes in the labour market, it is good to keep in mind something an experienced doctor said to me a couple of years ago. According to him, people who came into the reception in the 1970s were "from a different world" than today, but so was physicians' occupational culture and paradigm of mental ill-health. In this book, I set out to explore the change in a world that, in my view, has taken place at the interfaces of cultural change, the knowledge transformation and labour market transformation.

2

Mental vulnerability and the moving target of mental health

The perspective of mental vulnerability

I shall start my analysis with the concept of '*vulnus*'. This Greek concept means a wound. According to Hannah Arendt's (1998 [1958]) existentialism, every human being is vulnerable, and vulnerability is unique to the human condition. As relational beings, people are open to various influences in their social environments (Honkasalo, 2018). From the moment everyone is born, they start to act as a bodily being in a social world and are open to vulnerabilities (Lysaker, 2014). This perspective particularly stresses vulnerability as a key characteristic of the human existence. From this perspective a human is both an actor and a sufferer (Arendt, 1998 [1958]).

As a scientific concept, vulnerability emerged in the environmental sciences in reference to the impact of natural or economic disasters on human populations (Wisner and Luce, 1993; Virokannas et al, 2020). In addition, the concept is used in medicine and public health as an epidemiological term (Hutcheon and Lashewicz, 2014). Social researcher of law Jonathan Herring (2016) proposes that there are two main schools of thought, with the first emphasizing vulnerability as a universal human condition and the other focusing on certain people or groups as vulnerable. The identification of vulnerable populations has achieved wide popularity in social policy, social work, public health and applied psychology.

In my view, mental vulnerability is not primarily understood from the perspective of vulnerable groups in need of intensified psychological support and arsenals of mental protection (for example, elderly employees, young jobseekers and so on) and my intention is not to increase the stigmatization and pathologization often related to it (Zubin and Spring, 1977; Fawcett, 2009; Munro and Scoular, 2012). Most importantly, my approach to the mental vulnerabilities of our era aims to analyse a broader historical turn in the structural circumstances and social strategies of the subjects that have produced concern, a need for analyses and intentions of control related to a potentially vulnerable mental existence. Hence, my analysis is historical and social in nature, focusing on the phenomenon of mental vulnerability.

In this book, I draw on the idea of human openness and, at the same time, the social nature of human suffering in the analysis of the emergence of mentally troubled subjectivity. By studying the unique nature of human beings and their vulnerabilities during a considerable historical period in different occupational, public, scientific and political contexts, it is possible to identify how the transformation of culture and the change of the behavioural structure have moved us towards mental vulnerabilities. It also enables a better understanding of how the position of mental suffering and incapacity related to work has transformed during the change in work and work cultures. Thus, I focus on how the cultural emergence of new vulnerabilities among working-age people became possible and gained exceptional popularity in our historical era.

The concept of mental vulnerability points to the social and institutional nature of mental functioning, which is re-evaluated and redefined in various historically specific contexts. It stresses that mental wellbeing and psychological challenges are strongly embedded in temporally unique societal needs (for example, competencies and capacities at work) and normative standards (for example, adequate emotional expressions, favoured explanatory schemes). This view emphasizes the role of cultural and productive life-worlds in the formation of late modern psyche and capacity for work.

The concept of mental vulnerability is dual in nature: it situates mental vulnerabilities in cultural and economic arenas where the abilities and qualities of the working-aged are valued and labelled, and simultaneously points to people's historically changing abilities and a readiness to explain and narrate their subjectivity. This approach to vulnerability also signifies that I do not approach mental vulnerability as a sign of an insufficient level of individual resources or an automatic signal of weakness but as a part of social action that can also signify opportunities to express oneself and one's feelings. This means that mental vulnerability can be manifested both in the contexts of material scarcity and the contexts filled with abundant choices and options to fulfil one's subjective needs and objectives. The double-edged role of mental vulnerability includes both components of burdens and resources. In the critical analysis of current culture this leads to an interesting question: How have the potential changes in our behavioural codes, emotional coping strategies and ways of dealing with psychological hardships impacted the ways in which mental health frameworks have emerged and started to structure the challenges of work and the experiences of individuals?

I use distinct analytical frameworks in order to parse mental vulnerability. From a historical perspective, mental vulnerability stresses the historicity of mental challenges and the social codes of emotional life in different eras. On the socio-political level, mental vulnerability is produced and remade in the institutional practices and norms that regulate mental-health-related work abilities and disabilities. This manifests in practical solutions and categories offered to people in mentally challenging situations. Culturally, it is a continuous production of meanings, social relationships and shared identities in different social communities. On the economic level, it is a determined process of developing and identifying capacities for the delivery of material wealth and forms of capital which are important to the vitality of society. On the level of social behaviour, mental vulnerability is related to interaction, which helps to produce categories (classification), pinpoint relevant issues (power), communicate between people (interaction) and regulate our lives (management). In this book, I will particularly dissect the long-term labour-market-related and socio-cultural mechanisms that have jointly expanded the area, the role and significance of mental vulnerabilities as a characteristic of work, work-related wellbeing and the subject.

This approach does not deny the existence of mental health challenges and suffering among various working-age populations but critically analyses how numerous conceptual, institutional and subjectively meaningful approaches – manifested in concepts and practices related to stress, anxiety, depression and so on – became relevant and needed in our work and culture. In this manner, I also ask why the social and psychological space related to mental health issues at work have widened so much and why both workers and citizens have the tendency to increasingly apply these perspectives of mental vulnerability in their lives.

For the interpretation of this book, it is important to structure the difference between the concepts of mental vulnerability and mental health. Thousands of scientific publications have been published on the mental health of workers in occupational health sciences, psychology, epidemiology, medicine and other disciplines. Various large-scale studies have identified risk factors ranging from early childhood conditions (Negele et al, 2015) to personality (Klein et al, 2011), from genetic makeup (Demirkan et al, 2011) to poor cognitive reserve (Koenen et al, 2009), and more. Although these studies have provided information about the factors underlying an individual's mental health, the genetic, cognitive and even micro-social characteristics of individuals have not changed as considerably as the rise of mental vulnerabilities seems to indicate. Therefore, the broad question of the emergence of mental vulnerability remains intact. The transition towards mental vulnerability is taking place on the cultural, institutional and economic level of the society and influences the everyday challenges and core structures of social behaviour and emotional management while research and most interventions targeted on mental health take place on the individual or micro-social level, with little attention being paid to the structural transitions.

To illustrate the difference between mental health and vulnerability, I will provide an example from the field of life-course epidemiology, which has become popular among social epidemiologists and public health scientists as statistical techniques have improved, data registers have developed and cohorts have matured. When we examine mental health research, the important difference between life-course epidemiology and cultural/social research on mental vulnerability lies in the standpoint. The first one stems from individual life and mental health trajectories, while the second one focuses on shared 'cultural trajectories'. For instance, if we consider young employees, the epidemiological approach views the life course of a young person, its difficulties and risk factors that may adversely impact mental health if the past individual trajectory has been vulnerability-causing. From the cultural trajectory perspective, young persons are co-creators of a cultural trajectory as they share experiences with other people of their community, follow learned practices in the management of emotions, and base their behaviour on collective repertoires and value systems. The cultural trajectory perspective gains at least indirect support from history: some 50–60 years ago we had a very limited number of work-related mental health problems, or at least they were socially supressed and acted out differently. It is difficult to understand this transition using the life-course perspective and investigating mental health trajectories. Many researchers have also pointed out that the phenomenon of mental vulnerability can hardly be explained by the fact that over the past few decades, the labour market and the components of occupational health trajectories in Western countries have become more mentally burdensome than during previous historical periods (for example, early industrial societies) or indeed in contemporary developing economies (see Jones et al, 2001; Wainwright and Calnan, 2011).

From the perspective of mental vulnerability, we find a need to better understand social behaviours in mental health and gather information about the engines of mental vulnerability and the sources that are creating a need for psychological support. To achieve this purpose, we need studies that analyse how coping strategies, expectations, emotion codes, hegemonic knowledge structures, employee ideals, concepts of health, criteria of work ability and other crucial components affecting our collective understanding have changed and how this is reflected in our way of acting in terms of mental vulnerabilities. To understand the massive growth of mental vulnerabilities among working-age adults we need to focus our attention on the social nature of our being and how our socio-cultural relatedness is the basis for our social vulnerabilities.

The historical nature of social character

In their best-selling book, *The Lonely Crowd*, David Riesman and colleagues (1950) suggested that there are three types of social character: tradition-directed, inner-directed and other-directed. Their theory on social behavioural types suggested that human beings can be grouped into these three major types of social character. The tradition-directed people are orientated in the conventional ways of their ancestors. Inner-directed people turn to their own inner values and standards for guidance in their behaviour while other-directed persons depend upon the people around them to give direction to their actions (Kassarjian, 1962). In addition to Riesman and his colleagues, in the mid-1900s, some seminal social scientists (for example, Gerth and Mills, 1954; Whyte, 1956) analysed fascinatingly how the fundamental structure of the social character changes as societies and organizations change.

Although the theory is a child of its time, these ideas can capture something essential about the construction of mental vulnerability when it delves into the change in the soil of social behaviour. According to my interpretation, the social character refers to a social and emotional cornerstone attached to historical circumstances, whose basis of action change as society and the cultural environment change. For example, in Finland's agrarian society of the early 1900s, work, community and religion set frameworks for action and thinking, whereas the society of the early 2000s social behaviour is secularized, digitalized, and differentiated in the new way.

The character perspective incorporates the idea of the power of material operating conditions, the weight of culture and the importance of active agency. Social character constitutes a meso-level link between institutions and individuals (Shilling and Mellor, 2022). It describes the intersection in which mental vulnerabilities are enacted and constructed between changing manners and traditions, socio-economic frameworks, and the ideals and values of the period. The concept of social character is fundamental for social behaviour and identity, because idealized social characters represent exemplary behaviours for individuals and social groups. 'On the one hand they claim to describe social realities, and on the other they provide an opportunity for social self-understanding and ethical positioning' (Moser and Schlechtriemen, 2019). From my perspective, the social character framework provides a model for understanding the collective creation of ideal employees and meanings concerning normality and pathology within the context of changing work, work disability and occupational health. Our everyday micro-social circumstances entail various automatized and naturalized models of action and value structures which have changed over the decades. If we can capture these changes through historical, ethnographic and other materials we may understand more profoundly why the topic of mental health has become such a major issue in many affluent societies.

By analysing the historical formation of social character, this book examines mental vulnerability as an intimate part of action within the labour market and culture. Changes in the social character can be detected, for example, by looking at action strategies at work, ideal characteristics of employees or optimal ways of regulating emotions. My aim is to develop an analysis of how problems that are increasingly seen as mental health challenges are linked to the temporality of our social actions in the labour market and in our community, and how concepts such as health also take on new content as society and historical subjectivity change. This perspective calls for the inclusion of an active historical agency in the analysis. For instance, according to this view, 'determinants of mental ill-health' or 'psychosocial stressors' do not necessarily 'relate to' or 'associate with' lower social class or other conventional socio-economic indicators as we have learned in research on class inequalities, but they are merely perceived, enacted and communicated in relation with others in certain circumstances of work and other spheres of life (Olakivi, 2018). In this way, emotional codes within sub-cultures (for example, occupational groups) among other things define a threshold in which psychological, social and organizational challenges are produced through the prism of mental health. From this perspective, both mundane descriptions and views of professionals offer important information about the changing nature of vulnerabilities (for example, Shorter, 2013; Väänänen et al, 2019).

Within this theoretical framework knowledge on mental health, the solutions and beliefs associated with it and the social representations that explain its emergence are part of the construction of mental vulnerability. In turn, disabilities and health-related norms are related to the shared meaning defining criteria of good employees, and in that way, the supported as well as less favoured social character in labour markets. In line with these ideas, social theorists Chris Shilling and Philip Mellor (2022) have suggested that the tradition of character studies may be useful in building bridges between structural analyses and individual-oriented research. By analysing the standards and starting points of social activity through the social character metaphor, it is perhaps possible to get to grips with how we have a high level of material wellbeing at the population level, but at the same time a historically large number of forms of mental vulnerability. Thus, the analysis of the possibilities and repertoires of social characters representing different eras can open a view for understanding the current position of mental vulnerability (see also Shilling and Mellor, 2022).

An influential sociologist, Richard Sennett (Sennett, 1998) made a seminal analysis of the transition of the social character due to flexible capitalism and its behavioural requirements and scales of acting. Sennett analyses how our cultural and economic environment have deep impacts on our personal character (Sennett, 1998: 10). In this context, character is the ethical value we place on our own desires and on our relations to others. Character is a more encompassing term than its more modern offspring 'personality'. According to Sennett, flexible capitalism is searching for ways to destroy the evils of routine by creating more flexible institutions and models of action.

The practices of flexibility, however, focus mostly on the forces bending and shaping people (Sennett, 1998: 46). He analyses with a pessimistic tone: 'There is a question of corrosion of middle-class identity narrative and its meaningfulness' (Sennett, 1998: 122). He also connects the trap of flexibility with the long-term degrading of the middle classes in the Anglo-American economies, arguing that 'downward mobility among middle classes generates ambiguous and liminal conditions' (Sennett, 1998: 132; see also Ehrenreich, 1989). Overall, the view that people have gradually replaced an inner moral compass with organizational and interpersonal conformity has become popular among sociologists. In this new social order, social roles and identities that had once been institutionally provided now need to be found or constructed. In Sennett's analysis, these identities had become mostly situational and fleeting for strategic reasons because the long-term commitments no longer provide security and appropriate opportunities in market-driven capitalism.

Riesman and Sennett analysed the macro-level societal and labour market changes and how they are manifested in a behavioural constellation and coping strategies among working-age individuals. As Andrew Sayer (2020) has pointed out, Sennett studied the ethical value of the character and how it has gradually vanished and been replaced with a new flexible character, one that has started to navigate in the networks and changing circumstances caused by the neoliberal economical order. Assuming that structural change in the strategic and ethical field of social activity underlies the rise of mental vulnerability, linking the transitions of production with the management of psychological life and moral codes of behaviour is highly important in the analysis of mental vulnerabilities as socio-cultural phenomena. This analysis also attaches mental vulnerability to the history of Western subjectivity as the economy and the social structure of work have changed. Sennett's analysis suggests that the work-related commitments and attachments to workmates have impaired and led to a loss of trust towards others and a sense of meaning.

Partly in a similar way, in my analytical framework, the social character settles on a long historical trajectory in which being an employee and the structures that generate vulnerability change. However, instead of the transformation of the capitalist economy, a broader change in the norms of social character and the position of the psyche in work and culture are in focus. This choice also means an analysis of social opportunities and boundaries of action that extends beyond the labour market. To gain better insight into the surge of mental vulnerabilities among working-age adults from the 1960s to the 2020s, we need to look at the transitions of behavioural structures and possibilities of the social character in organizations and occupational health as well as in broader cultural and class environments. By analysing structural changes in social agency, it is possible to identify mechanisms that feed vulnerability manifested in various mental health pathologies and disability. This challenge with a historically changing character and its key concerns (for example, mental health disability) is largely an empirical question that falls between social sciences and psychology, but it also needs contributions from disciplines such as anthropology, history, epidemiology and critical psychiatry as well as a variety of other sciences (Sayer, 2020).

Simultaneously, a gradual change in the idea of vulnerability and in how we try to deal with it has occurred. In this way, the change of mental vulnerability is intertwined with the actual circumstances shaping the cavalcade of social characters as well as socially shared and temporally changing norms, morals and ideals. In order to understand the significant expansion of the social status of mental health in various contexts of work, it is important to focus on how the social character has changed in different parts of labour market and what kind of conditions the character types of different periods are based on. It is also important to recognize how characters and the vulnerabilities associated with them manifest prevalent cultural behavioural strategies and codes. It is valuable to note how some aspects or forms of character gain more institutional recognition and discursive space. In this way, it is also about power and the way it is used in different social fields.

Although this approach stresses the importance of historically unique meaning making and collective processes in creating vulnerabilities, it also stresses the role of economic and material conditions which often stimulate and/or create dynamics of mental vulnerability. Given this, the analytical focus on the historically conditional social character and its behavioural structure also enables the analysis of ostensibly paradoxical processes such as the development of materially wealthy labour market conditions and the parallel growth of mental health disabilities among younger generations of affluent economies. Thus, by linking the 'productive human' and 'cultural human' in the concept of social character, can provide new perspectives on why psychological work-related challenges are growing rapidly especially among young generations in current Western societies.

This book distances itself from theoretical models typical for occupational health research and many sciences studying work, such as work psychology, economic sociology and work-related social epidemiology. Instead, the analyses in this book are linked to many critical analyses made by numerous social scientists and cultural critics as they analyse work, agency and health. This can be seen in the references I make, for example, to individualisation, ideals of good workers and other cultural trajectories that have been part of the construction of vulnerability. This book would not be possible without the observations of social theorists, historians of work, investigators of medicalization and many others, who have made observations and presented alternative ideas about of mental health and its temporal and power-related nature.

Especially some social interactionists and theorists of dialogism have been important for how I understand the dynamic between the historical action and the social nature of humans. These approaches offer an alternative to traditional individualistic approaches in behavioural and social sciences. For instance, at the beginning of the 1900s American social psychologist and pragmatist George Herbert Mead (2015) was one of the pioneers of social psychology who theorized how we learn about ourselves and others through interaction with others (Smith and Hamon, 2012). If we apply Mead's conceptualization, we carry our cultural surroundings and social relationships as a 'generalized other' within ourselves. Similarly, Russian philosopher and literary critic Mikhael Bakhtin's (1981, 1993) theories of the dialogic nature of human subjectivity point out how we craft the reality around us by using shared language, dialogical interaction with others and by observing and understanding cultural contexts (Leiman, 1998; see Vygotsky, 1962; Bakhtin, 1981; Voloshinov, 1986).

According to interactionism and the tradition of dialogism, we both as professionals, researchers and lay persons formulate our views, express our thoughts and interpret feelings about ourselves and others in certain social and institutional settings. Within certain cultures, we intend to act properly with others who share similar emotional and social norms and ideals with us (see also Reay, 2005; Silvonen, 2015). One might even go further and suggest that instead of individuals, we are historically unique 'duoviduals' (my translation), as Finnish social psychologist Klaus Weckroth (2020) has formulated.

If we apply these ideas to mental vulnerability, it is always relational and takes place in certain socio-cultural circumstances. The relationality of mental vulnerability is a processual part of social behaviour that has several stakeholders, roles, norms, interests and institutional frameworks. Hence, mental vulnerability is meaningful only within some cultural interactive setting and should be analysed via those settings. At the heart of this book is the study of the historical frameworks of workers and other actors who build occupational health and rebuild the role of the psyche in the labour market (see Newton, 1998, 2009). For this reason, it has been important to focus on historical persons in their circumstances. How have they seen their situation? With what concepts? With what opportunities, status options, rules and prospects? How did they view their lives and life courses? What were the behaviours they saw as plausible given their social communities and social status? What was the understanding of mental health? How were different vulnerabilities related to their work and everyday living?

For this reason, the analyses are guided by two perspectives. First of all, we need to analyse the generation of mental vulnerabilities in real life circumstances in offices, factories, professional discussions, and so on, as well as in various institutional contexts and public forums where opinions, thoughts and emotions concerning desired work content and wellness at work are defined and manifested. Furthermore, the new epidemics of our time cannot be understood without systemically studying various organizational, institutional, scientific and professional arrangements that provide a structuring framework for vulnerability and conceptual interpretations. From this perspective, the mental health epidemic among the working-age population is not an etiological but historical and cultural research challenge. It also suggests that medical or psychological approaches and procedures can be considered as the prevailing systems related to current hegemonic culture that are increasingly surrounding our subjectivity and describe our intentions to manage its challenges. They provide an apparatus of structuring emotions and leave their mark on us as we interpret our own vulnerability and its status in our actions (Heidegger, 1962: 426).

According to this perspective, documents produced by employees, scientists, professionals and other institutional and non-institutional parties during a long timeline are likely to provide essential information on the emergence of mental vulnerability in late modern work. Due to the historically crafted nature of mental vulnerabilities, descriptions and remarks from different eras that describe typical occupational strains, behavioural tactics and observed alternatives for action can provide highly valuable information on the social transition associated with the emergence and normalization of current vulnerabilities. Therefore, magazine texts, occupational debates, professional observations, scientific publications and other materials that reflect how psycho-emotional challenges have been understood, framed and dealt with are relevant for my analysis.

The cultural nature of mental health understanding

Cultural differences can reveal important insights about the relational sense-making in occupational contexts and the dialogical understanding of work environment and wellbeing. I will give two examples from my previous studies which have had a cross-national comparative perspective. The first one comes from the European Working Conditions Survey that we reported for the Ministry of Social Affairs and Health in Finland in the early 2010s (Vartia et al, 2012). In the study we analysed the prevalence of gender discrimination in European countries stratified by gender and occupational status. To our surprise we found that it was not the well-educated women of the Northern European welfare countries who reported least gender discrimination in the EU, as could be expected. In contrast, according to survey responses, it was Portuguese blue-collar women who reported the least gender-related discrimination. This raised many questions related to the questionnaire method and the cultural specificity of the answers.

The second example of my scientific life comes from a cross-cultural study on the psychosocial working conditions and wellbeing I conducted with my colleagues among employees of a large-scale global industrial company using the same questionnaire in different countries (Väänänen et al, 2005). From the beginning, we knew that all employees of the company had rather similar and standardized working conditions in the operating countries. However, we were quite surprised when we saw the results of the analyses: in contrast to other industrial employees working in other countries, the Chinese perceived themselves as considerably autonomous at work.

I argue that neither Portuguese blue-collar employees nor Chinese industrial employees had a privileged position compared to the workers in other countries. I rather suggest that the low-educated Portuguese blue-collar female employees of the early 2000s had less cultural knowledge and were less oriented towards debates of gender equality and discrimination than women in Northern Europe. Formulated in a more theoretical way, their prevalent social character forms (for example, female blue-collar standards and role models) and value systems (for example, the significance of gender equity) did not prioritize these types of expressions and even regarded them as rather irrelevant in their daily organizational life. Hence, the results did not indicate a low level of discrimination among them. In turn, in Chinese work culture, workers' autonomy was not a number one priority in the early 2000s, but rather external discipline was emphasized. When an employee was situated in Westernized working conditions requiring more autonomous behaviours the 'cultural context of autonomy' stood out and high levels of autonomy were reported. The situation was different compared to Western employees who have a macro-culture stressing the importance of individual integrity and autonomous decision-making. Both observations are central in terms of culturally and historically embedded agency.

Taken together, the dialogical character is manifested in our views and interpretations of our environment. Without understanding the culturally meaningful social behaviours, emotional codes and expectations within which a social subjectivity is embedded, it is quite challenging to develop a valid analytical perspective concerning employees' social action.

An influential cultural critic, Raymond Williams (1961) has formulated that 'everyone living through a period would have something which no later individual can wholly recover'. An existentialist philosopher, Charles Guignon (1990: 109) has vocabularized the historicity of humans using a narrative approach: 'Life-stories only make sense against the backdrop of possible story-lines opened by our historical culture.' From the perspective of structural anthropology, Claude Levi-Strauss (2009 [1955]) has argued that individual cultural practices could only be made sense of by looking at the relationship with other practices in the same culture. All these formulations coming from different branches of science point to historically specific behavioural and emotional structures embedded in demands of working life, ideals of an era and each person's own social context. Hence, to understand the troubled nature of mental existence in the early 21st century, it is necessary to rethink what it is like to be a person today and how we as social actors see ourselves and others (for example, people, institutions, researchers) within these historical practices. Using Levi-Strauss's words, we have to study cultural practices (for example, habits, opportunities, means) that are available for us as historical subjects in work and elsewhere (see also Suzman, 2021). Thus, to observe the uniqueness of favoured social perceptions and peculiarities, comparisons between different cultures or data accumulated within the same society over a long period of time could be used. Historical materials can reveal, for instance, how similar issues were placed in the earlier contexts of work.

This dialogical perspective requires examining how various vulnerabilities are intended to be managed as a professional, organizational, academic and political challenge. It carries the double meaning of subjectivity as both the 'first-personness' of consciousness (being a subject *of* experience) and the conditioning of that consciousness by our society, culture and time (being subject *to* power, authority or influence) (Tafarodi, 2013). In the critical view, it is crucial to rethink the current hegemonic understanding of subjectivity (Geertz, 1973, 1983; Biehl et al, 2007). For instance, guidelines related to coping in stressful situations and recommendations for individuals (for example, stress management) need a critical analysis as they typically reproduce social norms concerning individual's responsibility and leave the underlying structures that create stressful subjects outside the analysis.

In the late 20th century and early 21st century, there have been several structural transformations in our culture and production which have stimulated the emergence of new languages and institutional ways of understanding subjectivity. In the labour market, there are numerous classification systems, processes and objectives organized around mental health. Consequently, being a dialogical subject in the context of work and health has considerably changed. To understand this crucial change, we need to systematically collect and analyse information produced by employees, professionals and other crafters of vulnerability. This approach also differs from commonly used occupational health models. For instance, most widely used theoretical models of psychosocial occupational health, such as the job strain model (Karasek, 1979; Karasek and Theorell, 1990), effort-reward model (Siegrist, 1996) and demands/resources model (Bakker and Demerouti, 2007), approach the workplace as a measurable work environment, composed of health-promoting or health-deteriorating 'determinants', 'risks' or 'resources' that can be assessed using a set of questions. On the one hand, these models capture essential aspects of current work and pinpoint important psychosocial issues in the level of the observable immediate surroundings. On the other hand, these approaches tend to frame employees as 'informants' who report their observations of their surrounding conditions and are affected by 'work conditions'. This epistemic choice inevitably excludes the 'cultural actor' from the analysis. This framing is problematic if we want to get a more detailed picture of the development of mental vulnerability and the long-term change in its status at work.

One of the extremes of subject-eliminating research is represented by epidemiological approaches in which psychosocial exposure is being inferred from objective occupational exposure matrices. These matrices are often based on an assessment by experts and researchers of average occupational exposures (chemical, physical, biological and psychosocial agents) for a list of jobs. This information is usually coded according to some established classification system and places the employee somewhere in the exposure indicator (Choi, 2020). In this way, exposure to mental illness can be assessed without any information from the subject and the risk can be evaluated by looking at the statistical data. In this way, research is based on the idea that both the 'surroundings' and an individual's 'mental health' can be measured with validated instruments and the connections between them can be described with correlations and risk relations. From the perspective of mental vulnerability, it is necessary to ask how a historically transformative subject, with its desires, goals and learned manners, fits into this thought pattern.

Both historical research of work and the history of ideas show that classifications and activities in the field of mental health have varied at different times (Porter, 1997; Väänänen et al, 2014; Jenkins, 2015). Instead of external measurable risks, such perspectives point to a change in both the fundamental structure of work and the socio-emotional practices related to employees' vulnerability. Overall, these contrasts illustrate the long distance between the views of the natural sciences and social/humanistic studies in terms of mental vulnerability. However, they also suggest that research of mental health among working-age individuals would benefit from the social research of human vulnerability.

The moving target of mental health

In his classic study, social psychologist Kenneth Gergen (1973) stresses that most of the processes falling into the social domain are dependent on social dispositions and characteristics subject to modifications over time (Gergen, 1973: 317–318). This understanding emphasizes the difference between the 'indifferent kinds' studied within natural science and the 'interactive kinds' witnessed in social science (Collingwood, 1946; Hacking, 1999: 108; Connelly and Costall, 2000). Gergen emphasizes that the methods and concepts change over time in interactive cultural contexts and, at the same time, the objects that research tries to understand also change. Partly in a similar way, Ian Hacking (1999: 114) has framed social sciences and psychology as the study of 'a moving target' because these studies 'interact' with the social 'objects' we are trying to observe. If we think that the mental vulnerabilities of our historical period have roots in our social life and our social conditions that shape our understanding, it is important to study these characteristics of our time. This view means that vulnerabilities we discuss and observe in our societies and labour market are continuously affected by various scientific findings, professional debates, good clinical practices and political intervention proposals that are made. Research and professional practices on burnout, stress and depression 'move their target'.

Not only social and psychological scientific knowledge influence our understanding and self-understanding of employees, supervisors, health professionals and other stakeholders, but conventional media, social media and other information channels also produce reinterpretations and narrations that 'move the target'. In this vein, mental vulnerabilities have a rather distinctive nature compared to traditional health challenges that are typically open to biological/physiological examination and do not change to the same extent while we name, classify and try to manage them. Simultaneously, the professional cultures and classification systems capturing mental vulnerabilities do not remain intact but are merely affected by societal transitions related to ideal subjects and general views on troublesome characteristics (Väänänen et al, 2012, 2019).

If we want to understand the emergence of mental vulnerability at work, canonized approaches based on the separation of the individual and the explanation of the individual state of mental health and work disability tend to lead to dead ends. Instead, it becomes important to examine the transition of socio-historical forms of social character, social knowledge concerning this character and the transformation of mental vulnerability as a kind of by-product. As philosopher Rosi Braidotti (2019: 56) has formulated, this task is not just a scientific endeavour: 'In the absence of an adequate understanding of subjectivity, the very possibility of an ethical and political project that would enable us to come to terms with paradoxes and challenges of our times is quite simply undermined.' Social conditions are entangled and embodied in human subjectivity and therefore subjectivity needs to be understood and analysed from how people live their lives (Teo, 2023).

Mental vulnerabilities make sense in contexts where people of the same culture have shared meanings (for example, the importance of mental health), moral/ethical codes (for example, mental care of oneself) and institutional know-how (for example, professional channels of solution). Social character formulations we employ as historical subjects always build meanings, codes of conduct and knowledge on actions that can support the psyche. From the historical perspective, we have certain dramaturgical aspects of our character that are prevalent and successful during some historical periods which may not make sense in the social scenery of some other period. The view on historical and culturally adaptive and structuralized character that has certain behavioural schemas and forms of narrative and habitual ways for dealing with emotional self-management approaches the research work by Norbert Elias (1978, 1991, 1994) and Erving Goffman (1961). In his studies, Elias particularly emphasized the social embeddedness and consistency of our manners and emotional management. He analysed how our behavioural codes and emotional control have evolved over centuries and how some behaviours that were considered normal in pre-modern societies gradually became intolerable and morally avoidable as societies transferred towards modern civilizations. Goffman, in turn, studied people in their micro-social contacts and stressed how they learn and use everyday 'scripts' and interpret social frameworks to behave properly in the social arenas of our society. These analyses emphasize the importance of cultural ethos and morality for human subjectivity and how societal macro-processes influence the structure of the subject's mental self-understanding and emotional management. In this dynamic between the structure and the subject, employees learn and adapt to behave according to the 'feel of the game' (Albrecht, 2015: 602–604).

Because of the historical and social nature of mental vulnerability we should not so much study concepts similar to physical objects, like 'age groups', 'work', 'mental health', 'depression' and 'work disability', but instead look at normal behaviours, opinions and ideals of workers in different positions, of experts with various institutional roles, of labour market bodies with certain interests, of medical authorities as gatekeepers of mental health, of organizational management and so on. From this point of view, we have various social agents who craft mental vulnerabilities, relay views and facts about them, and relocate the position of mental capacity/strain in the social order. Historically speaking they are 'moving the target', using Hacking's expression.

Most importantly for social studies, we have the possibility to look at the formulations, expectations, options and social arrangements where vulnerability is crafted, understood, managed and modified over a long period of time. As Finnish sociologist Risto Heiskala (1994) has portrayed the Goffmanian spirit, we should view people as 'human beings in given moments' and analyse them within their temporal circumstances and habitual social positions available and desired (Thoits, 1989).

My general approach could be defined as a defamiliarization method (Braidotti, 2019: 19). By focusing on long-term changes, I aim to go beyond current frameworks and prevalent discourses and view social behaviour and the position/character of mental vulnerability in different times and historical contexts. From the ontological perspective, the mental vulnerabilities of our era can be viewed as an intimate part of a renewing and redefined subject (Semetsky, 2008). It can be thought that in our empirical studies, we analyse 'little movements' between the past, present and the future which have provoked a gradual new subject formation, including new understanding about humans at work as well as their mental vulnerabilities.

The case of Finland

Many historical transitions analysed in this book are shared across Western countries and working-age people of these societies. Technological change, urbanization, deindustrialization, the turn to service sector jobs, the feminization of the workforce, and the medicalization and liberalization of the labour markets are among the shared characteristics which have affected workers and work organizations across many countries. Probably due to shared social change and cultural backgrounds, elements of mental health crises have similarities between countries. This book uses a large set of scientific sources from various studies conducted mainly in Western countries that have experienced similar mental challenges. However, the elementary part of the empirical work for this book has been prepared in Finland.

Unlike in most Western countries, the Finnish economy was heavily based on agriculture and forestry until the 1950s. For instance, in the early 1950s, it was about 50 years behind the industrial development of the Swedish economy (Hannikainen and Heikkinen, 2006). Over the past 70 years, Finland has rapidly transformed from an agricultural society into an industrial society, and then into a late modern knowledge-intensive society. From the 1960s onwards, major demographic changes took place as working-age people started to move from rural settings to cities in bids to find employment in the new industrial and service sectors.

This drastic structural shift, accompanied throughout by changes in the level of education, were reflected in overall conditions of work and standards of living (Fellman, 2008; Sutela and Lehto, 2014). In the 1970s most employees had received only a basic level of education and were still rooted in the countryside. According to one of the oldest nationally representative working life surveys in Europe, in 1977 about 10 per cent of Finnish employees had a university degree, while by 2018 their share was 46 per cent (Sutela et al, 2019). The transition pointed to considerable changes in people's work practices and cultural outlooks. For instance, in 1984, 17 per cent of Finnish employees used information technology in their work, whereas in 2018 the corresponding rate was 91 per cent. During the same time, the possibilities to develop oneself at work increased considerably. In 1984, 28 per cent of employees reported that they had good opportunities to develop themselves, while in 2018 this had increased to 45 per cent.

A dramatic decline of low-skill jobs in agriculture and heavy industry took place between the 1960s and 1990s and there was a sharp increase in more knowledge-based work between the 1980s and 2010s (Pyöriä et al, 2005; Väänänen et al, 2016). In a range of studies, it is now documented that what is sometimes referred to as the 'golden era' of the Finnish wage worker, marked by material development, started to crumble from the 1980s onwards as the result of the cumulative impacts of the ever-intensifying forces of globalization, economic deregulation and automatization (Siltala, 2007; Bergholm and Bieler, 2013). When compared to other European countries and contexts (notably, the UK), most Finnish state welfare institutions survived these transitions in a relatively robust condition, although at the same time, neoliberal market ideology influenced Finnish occupational culture (Julkunen, 2003). There was a noticeable reconfiguration of collective institutions and their relations whereby earlier conventions rooted in political collectivism were partly eroded and were substituted in favour of a new emphasis on the pursuit of self-development, self-actualization and on the need for individual flexibility (Boltanski and Chiapello, 2007; Skeggs, 2011). Employees were increasingly required to develop and display 'resilience', 'flexibility' and 'productivity'; and often, this was accompanied by further pressures being placed on them to demonstrate an ongoing and ready willingness to adapt to new times (Kuokkanen et al, 2013).

These changes were accompanied by considerable transitions in the types of health problems that were set for treatment within the occupational health service and healthcare in general. The prevalence of chemical and physical hazards declined while various psychosocial exposures and needs for work stress management were identified (Kauppinen et al, 2013; Kinnunen-Amaroso and Liira, 2014). The proportion of cardiovascular diseases and injuries declined at the same time as there was an increase in mental health concerns. In the 1990s and the 2000s, the number of sickness absence spells due to mental disorders more than doubled and the use of antidepressant drugs grew fivefold (Järvisalo et al, 2005). Currently, the majority of disability benefits are granted for mental disorders (Nyman and Kiviniemi, 2018) and mental disorders compose the largest reason for longer sickness absences (Blomgren and Perhoniemi, 2022).

Our datasets provide versatile insights into how the labour market transition, the new composition of the workforce, new work requirements and the change of employee ideals modified the approaches towards mental vulnerabilities and the role of the psyche as an element of working capacity. These macroeconomic adjustments and cultural transitions were accompanied by organizational changes that left large numbers of people more prone to forms of mental exhaustion and distress. Public discussions on chronic stress, anxiety, burnout and depression became gradually more common, but so did numerous subjective reflections of work and wellbeing.

This historical turn also signified that occupational healthcare practitioners were left responding to ever increasing problems relating to the employees' subjective challenges (Lehtonen and Koivunen, 2010). The 'old tools' that applied to the health problems of Finland's 'golden era' (for example, physical examinations, stethoscopes, X-rays and so on) were increasingly made redundant by new psychological and organizational challenges.

To summarize, the Finnish society, culture and labour market provide an internationally interesting 'case country' for studying the surge of mental vulnerability in a context of rapid societal change. The generations of employees as well as other social agents who have experienced and lived the transition provide the main empirical material for this book. Their descriptions, narratives, remarks and analyses have been highly valuable but also controversial datasets in the construction of this book. Subjective accounts and interpretations are coloured by contextual shades and highly different perspectives often emerge when the occupational, organizational and historical context changes. However, I believe that only thorough materials covering a sufficiently lengthy historical period and a variety of data sources can provide an adequate basis for the analysis of mental vulnerability among the working-age population. Luckily, other researchers have also at least partly dealt with similar challenges. The next three chapters mainly draw from their work.

3

The vulnerability of work

There are varying approaches that link the surge of mental weariness and uneasiness at work with distinctive transitions in society. To clarify social scientific research on the emergence of mental health challenges and concerns among the working-aged, in this and the next chapter (Chapter 4) I have classified the analytical frameworks into different approaches that have been most often applied. These contain alternate standpoints and reasoning as well as differentiated views on the nature of mental vulnerabilities among late modern individuals. In this chapter I will focus on work-based frameworks.

The *first approach* highlights the role of the increasing emotional, social and cognitive demands of work that arise from globalization, growing competition, and strains caused by customer flows and information intensity. The argument stresses the adverse impact of burdening psychological, social and organizational demands on mental health in the context of late capitalism (for example, Green, 2006; Tausig and Fenwick, 2011a; Boxall and Macky, 2014). The *second approach* focuses on the decline and inflation of employees' position and standard employment relationship, which are linked to efforts to improve labour market efficiency and increasing demands of flexibility since the 1970s. According to this reasoning, critical shifts in the modes of production and the restructuring of organizations have generated economic displacement and organizational upheavals. Consequently, emotional despair and mental ill-health has spread, especially in declining industries and the newly disadvantaged classes of the labour market often labelled as 'precarious' (for example, Charlesworth, 2000; Williams, 2003; Standing, 2011).

Burdening of work

The fundamental basis for wellbeing is often associated with material and psychological resources. Work seems to have a highly ambivalent role from this perspective as it is portrayed both as a source of burden and personal/economic fulfilment both in research and public discussions. In general, changes in work conditions seems to have created new mentally challenging environments/cultures and provoked a surge in mental vulnerability. In this chapter, I will present how the research on work carries strong assumptions about the core source of mental vulnerability and the nature of the transition.

In the industrial sociology of the 1970s, labour process theory produced an account of how economic and political processes affected the quality of work (Tausig and Fenwick, 2011a: 56). In *Labour and Monopoly Capital*, Harry Braverman (1974) challenged the basic assumption made by Clark Kerr et al (1962), Daniel Bell (1973) and many others that the introduction of new, increasingly automated technologies would lead to upgrading workers' skills and well-being. In contrast, he estimated that under capitalism, mechanized and automated technologies would lead to deskilling or degradation of labour. The results were not only greater productivity with lower labour costs, but also greater managerial control over the production process. According to this argument, the transition had a considerable impact on the ways employees were treated and the psychological burden of work was increased. In the sociological research, the control of work processes was viewed as a central issue, unbalanced power structures were criticized and collective labour protection was called for. Thus, the concern about the harmfulness of monotonous factory work, once raised by Karl Marx and illustrated by Charlie Chaplin's film *Modern Times* (1936), arose in the 1970s in several countries. Indeed, the change in the status of factory work and the growth of modern organizations increased the need for work psychological knowledge and the desire to manage stress at work scientifically.

Another important step in the analysis of economic and work sociology was taken in the 1980s when Scott Lash and John Urry (1987) described an erosion of established ways of organizing and managing capitalism in *The End of Organized Capitalism*. In their view, the German-type industrial corporation became increasingly outdated, as ownership was more often dominated by financial institutions concerned with short-term 'shareholder value'. Anti-Keynesian perspectives became a flood in the early 1980s as progressivism and state-ism were rolled back, especially in the disorganization in the Anglo–American economies. 'The term "big bang" is apposite to capture this break as capitalism "disorganizes"' (Lash and Urry, 2013). Lash and Urry analysed the fragmentation of the national paradigm and its displacement by global neoliberalism, which reached countries like Finland in the 1980s as a form of 'casino economy'. According to many macro-level researchers of work, this caused considerable changes in the ways work was organized, managed and led (Julkunen, 2008). Robert Castells (1996) summarized it as a conflict between free flexibility and organized local regulation: the further globalization progressed, more evident has become the contrast between the free flow of capital and mobility and the inflexibility of labour contracts.

Many social scientists have analysed that the process of flexible capitalism (for example, Kjaerulff, 2015) was part of the surge of a 'risk society' emerging from a volatile environment (for example, Beck, 1992) and the rise of the 'network society' characterized by mutual interdependencies and market-driven globalization (Castells, 1996). According to this interpretation, the collective power of workers was weakened, and the negotiation capacity and know-how diminished. Market economies penetrated work organizations and employees' lives without institutional buffering mechanisms (Julkunen, 2008).

However, although there have been tendencies to reduce collective bargaining and state-level organizing of work, Finland and many other countries have not abandoned the national regulation of labour relations (Julkunen, 2008: 63). However, critical researchers of the Nordic labour market have also questioned this Nordic welfare mantra and asked whether skills-based labour management constitutes the foundation of the Nordic business model anymore. For instance, Finnish sociologist Markku Sippola (2012) has argued that in Finland deregulation and market-driven capitalism have led to deskilling and new flexibility requirements. This is not only the reality in the case of the lower tier of the labour market, but also with respect to white-collar workers. In some interpretations this tendency has converted the highly educated classes into a new type of proletariat, as their work has intensified so significantly and been filled with non-legitimate tasks and self-monitoring (for example, Carey, 2007; Levä, 2021).

This analytical perspective basically states that Harry Braverman's (1974) labour process theory still holds, and a major transition has occurred as the control of workers has also spread to new labouring classes characterized by high education, interactive work and knowledge intensity. This transition has been interpreted as 'an invasion of the periphery to the core' (Kunda and Ailon-Souday, 2006: 210). In many work organizations, working conditions that were once typical of peripheral employees are shared by core employees of the labour market. This interpretation is similar to that of Saskia Sassen's (1998: 147) notion of an overall tendency towards 'casualization of the employment relation' that has spread across the labour markets and to the high-end jobs as well.

From the perspective of mental vulnerability and the workplace, the main question in this tradition is how work is controlled and how much power employees have in terms of their work content, work pace and timing, amount of work, organization of work, and other key aspects of the work process. At the meso level of work organizations and micro level of individual employees, this perspective raises the topic of job control and external job demands. Some of these ideas have been operationalized in the tradition of occupational and psychosocial epidemiology. One of the most prominent conceptions in this area, 'the job strain model' (or 'job demand/control model'), stresses the importance of a healthy balance between job control and job demands (Karasek, 1979). In this work stress model, 'job demands', or quantitative and qualitative constrictions, were opposed by the calming protective resources of work, 'job control'. 'High strain jobs' are characterized by low control but high demands, a combination which is regarded as the most detrimental for the mental and physical health of employees. In this way, this model translates the ideas of macro-level sociological theories concerning deskilling and the corrosive impact of control into the concept of occupational exposure. For more than 40 years, this approach has been empirically tested in hundreds of studies in dozens of countries. However, according to recent meta-analyses and reviews, the job demand/control model has received modest empirical support as a predictor of employees' mental health and psychological wellbeing (Häusser et al, 2010; Madsen et al, 2017).

It is well-known that work has not remained the same between the 1970s and 2020s and countries differ considerably. From the context of information-intensive work (Väänänen and Toivanen, 2018; Väänänen et al, 2020), occupational class (Choi et al, 2015) and cultural difference (Schaufeli, 2017), universal work stress theories like the job strain model can be justly criticized. For instance, low control over one's work in the 'industrial sense' of the 1970s is no longer the main issue in many jobs, but the question of self-organizing and the management of own agency is increasingly essential. The content-related (for example, knowledge jobs) and cultural (for example, fewer hierarchies) transition in work also has signified a considerable change in the behavioural constellation of what it means to be a worker. The mindset of employees has transformed as the work process has changed from pre-organized mechanical production to socially complex immaterial production characterized by strong social dependencies (Väänänen et al, 2020). The importance of autonomous agency has increased, which is manifested in concepts such as self-development and psychological meaningfulness. In addition, the role of emotional and social skills has become more pronounced as interactive, communication-driven and consumer-oriented work has occupied more space in the occupational structure. This historical change has left several marks in occupational health by changing the stress-provoking monotonous structure of work towards new types of multi-location work and interdependencies that frame the structural conditions of being an employee. They have also stimulated various debates and studies on work–family interface, work/family conflict and other equivalent topics that are directly related to the increasing negotiation and overlapping between key spheres of life (Grzywacz et al, 2008; Michel et al, 2011).

Although simple linear models (for example, higher control > higher mental wellbeing) may be attractive in their way of parsing, they may be poor guidelines for developing organizational wellbeing and understanding of mental vulnerabilities in today's labour market. For instance, knowledge work and various forms of hybrid work call attention to the social framework and systemic nature of work (Väänänen et al, 2020).

Similar to the idea of Karasek's model, socio-epidemiological mental health research also places the well-being/nausea of the psyche of employees largely within the framework of work stressors and psychosocial exposure. In this context, the social inequalities of health are attributed to the accumulation and unharmonious distribution of stressful work characteristics (Marmot and Wilkinson, 2006). The definition by American health sociologists Mark Tausig and Rudy Fenwick illustrates the elementary idea of this approach as follows:

> We couple the argument that health disparities emerge because of the social patterning of stress exposure with the argument that the various structural arrangements in which individuals are embedded determine the stressors they encounter in a concrete social context, work. We posit a specific mechanism that links social inequality to labour market participation that in turn leads to jobs with stressful characteristics and subsequent distress or disorder. We therefore argue that the proper study of the relationship between social inequality and stress/distress should include the specification of specific structural arrangements such as work that become the proximal source of exposure to stressors. (Tausig and Fenwick, 2011a: 16)

This quotation reflects widely distributed arguments concerning the formation of mental health among employees and the inequality between different employee groups. It proposes that mental health problems are produced by various work-related structural arrangements and inequalities between employee groups. In this constellation, there are objective environmental and social characteristics that cause health-related adversity among employees. Furthermore, it suggests that these arrangements form stressors and this epidemiological ground can be approached using adequate research instruments and statistical techniques. This approach offers a science-based view that these stressors are exposures that can cause mental health problems and create a basis of inequality related to mental health in society. Hence, individuals are exposed to psychosocial/emotional exposures to different levels and therefore have a different risk of vulnerability.

Here we need to pause for a while as these assumptions also compose scientific knowledge on current 'psychosocial' occupational health, and thousands of studies on work-related wellbeing and mental ill-health are based on this kind of theorization. If these arguments are followed, we are surrounded by various virus-like stressors and some of us are more exposed to these damaging stress-viruses than others. In this way, mainstream occupational stress research, the psychosocial research of work and partly also the research of socio-economic inequalities at work have transferred medical modelling and exposure-outcome thinking to social and occupational environment of working-age populations. This shift has meant the birth of a peculiar scientific framework for the research of mental vulnerability and the differences of mental vulnerabilities at work. The approaches propose that 'key factors' and 'mechanisms' are mainly observable in the environment while the role of social agents as active subjects is limited to personality/ social status traits or micro-social climates. Hence, studies measure individuals as 'optimistic', 'elderly', 'women', 'manual workers' and so on, but their agencies, habitual forms of psychological coping, values, priorities and overall social behaviour related to psycho-emotional challenges are not placed in their cultural contexts and social history. Individuals are expected to react biologically and psychologically to the external stressors they experience.

A more structural alternative to psychosocial perspectives has been offered by British economist Francis Green (2006). He points out that in the market liberal societies, such as the UK, increased competition and efficiency requirements have promoted the need for employers to exercise greater control over the size of their workforce; to be able to 'hire and fire at will' to respond to fluctuations in demand and to increase efficiency through corporate 'downsizing' or 're-engineering'. These transitions have been manifested in employment legislation since the early 1980s and the rise of the fixed-term contract and consultancy work in the UK and US. According to Green (2006), it was actually the redistribution of insecurity towards the increasing middle classes that has accounted for its high media profile and fuelled various forms of mental health epidemics (for example, work stress) in the early 2000s. This also leads to the idea of how the destabilization of the middle class potentially began to produce mental health epidemics.

Interestingly, in one of our own Finnish interview studies, occupational health physicians understood many of their patients to be experiencing mental health problems because of increasing work pressures and drastic organizational changes especially since the 1980s (Wilkinson and Väänänen, 2021):

> It was those big mergers (in the 1980s and early 90s) in the sectors where people had a belief that once you get in and start there you can stay until you retire. Suddenly, the firms started to fall and merge. Those were quite shocking situations. I remember a social event when a bank employee told that it was like spouse's death when her bank went bankrupt. People had a strong workplace identity and all of a sudden they were told that this is closed and does not exist anymore. That was a time when I realized that I take care of communities not individuals, [and this includes both] their worries and their despair. After that the profit-making objectives were introduced, and employees of the banks became salespersons. Once, a long time ago, employees had been recruited because of good handwriting skills … how could the same persons now transform themselves into efficient top sellers? … The demands became intolerable for the psyche. Of course, some

individuals took it on and managed to float somehow, but some took it hard. (Female doctor born in 1961, started practising in 1980s)

In line with these findings, health sociologists David Wainwright and Michael Calnan (2002) argue that the subjective fear of job loss may have risen sharply, causing workers to intensify their labour in order to avoid dismissal or other negative individual consequences. In this macroeconomic context of labour market change, psychological effects are likely, and they can be manifested in anxiety, uncertainty and frustration. This observation about the changing economy and work points to a highly important structural change in the map of mental vulnerabilities: a considerable increase of middle-class occupations as well as the rise of psychological demands and psychology-driven cultures since the late 1970s in the growing middle classes.

During the two first decades of the 21st century, work intensification has been found to be a new emerging psychosocial risk across Europe (Brun and Milczarek, 2007). As a concept, work intensification often refers to circumstances in which the work demands exceed an employee's ability to cope with them, for example, tight deadlines, high-speed work, pace induced by external factors and long working hours. There has been some evidence that cultures with long working hours have become more prevalent in some EU countries (Żołnierczyk-Zreda et al, 2012), but if long-term trends over the past 60 years are evaluated, the working hours have declined considerably according to available pan-European data sources. It seems that the new structure of the labour market and the rule of flexible capitalism has produced more pressures that exceed employees' mental health resources, but they are not easily approached using objective measures such as working time.

To understand the interrelationship between labour market transitions and mental vulnerability, we need more information on how subjects view their work situation and how the relationship towards work may have changed in the long run. An interesting observation is offered by the Finnish Working Life Barometer (Keyriläinen, 2021), which measures the changes in subjective experiences related to the meaningfulness of one's job among the Finnish workforce. According to the barometer, the meaningfulness of work declined throughout the 2000s and 2010s. It has been argued that through the adoption of American standards, companies have damaged the moral contract between employers and employees, according to which loyalty, security and decent treatment is expected from the employer as a reward for work efforts of the employees (Alasoini, 2012).

There are strong predispositions in research on work to link macroeconomic changes with individual accounts made by questionnaire respondents, seducing the researcher to draw causal assumptions between neoliberal market regimes and people's declining psychological wellbeing. Working life surveys are culturally and historically contextual, measured at a particular time point often using self-rated measures (for example, feelings of hurry, level of psychological demands and so on). Work is regarded as a measurable entity including environmental, social and psychological factors impacting the subjects regardless of their background. People are conceptualized as 'informants' who can provide data on their circumstances, work features, health, and other key dimensions of work and mental wellbeing more or less objectively without the cultural burden of temporality and locality.

This leads, in turn, to three problems for the analysis of the emergence of mental vulnerabilities in Western societies. First, studies are inclined towards reductionism: mental vulnerability is understood as determined by macroeconomic changes and its declining trends. The variability in social action in relation to vulnerability plays a secondary role. Second, the research has a strong tendency towards universalism: workers are typically regarded as psychological and biological entities having rather similar 'human characteristics', needs and sources of wellbeing. Historical variations in subjectivity (for example, aspects of the historical social character) related to shifts in generations and values are not regarded as a key issue. Finally, an understanding of mental health characterizes most studies: depression, anxiety, exhaustion and burnout are principally understood as concepts that can be approached and evaluated using standardized measures and/or diagnostic categories. In other words, the political character and the socio-cultural nature of mental vulnerabilities remains mostly unexplored.

All in all, within this research context mental vulnerabilities of work have been attributed to the inner transitions of the labour market and the economy. There is no doubt that excessive work demands or working hours have detrimental mental health impacts on a population scale: seeking short-term profits, efficiency and a lower cost structure have inconvenient side-effects that are often manifested in an individual's mental wellbeing. However, the importance of objective methods and the golden standards of natural sciences (for example, randomized control, prospective modelling, methodological individualism) typical for social epidemiology and applied psychology often leave societal and cultural changes affecting employees beyond their scope. In turn, sociological studies on work easily lead to overgeneralizations in terms of flexible capitalism, the intensification of work and how these processes are reflected in patterns of mental suffering in different groups of employees.

In order to understand the psychological vulnerability that has recently emerged, it would be essential to delve into social and organisational structures at the interfaces between changing work and changing historical subjects. The interpretation offered by work sociologist Raija Julkunen (2008: 60) serves as an example. According to her, the feelings of uncertainty and insecurity that are often discussed in current studies on work do not directly reflect the real threats that occur at a given moment. If we exclude direct global health threats, working-aged people in most parts of Europe are very well protected against starvation, diseases, occupational accidents and homelessness when viewed on a historical and global scale. She interprets the feeling of insecurity to stem from the imbalance between culturally produced expectations of security and the opportunities in society to respond to these expectations. These observations are not only important in terms of an understanding of insecurity, but they can also be applied to a broader framework of work and vulnerability.

If today's working-age population evaluate their situation from the personal perspective, they are likely to use different criteria and different perceptual/conceptual frameworks than past generations due to culturally produced expectations. For this reason, self-reported symptoms or observations on the features of work are not objective reflections of the circumstances in society and the labour market. For instance, subjective and self-reported perceptions of work stress, psychological distress, uncertainty and hurry are formed within a certain framework of historical possibilities and storylines. Therefore, a high prevalence of uncertainty could be more likely in societies that emphasize the importance of security, prediction and manageability (Julkunen, 2008). Similarly, a high level of work stress or anxiety may reflect how much importance is given to work-related emotions in public and professional discussions, to what extent subjective feelings are valued in work and to what extent they are seen as part of health.

Precarious work as an engine of vulnerability

An important strand in the social sciences has focused on the alleged growth of mental health problems in certain populations that are more open to destructive forces of global capitalism. In the background of this research tradition lies the economy-driven transition from a stable period of growth to the less stable and less predictable period of uncertainty and economic decline since the end of 1900s. The research focus is on the forced transition of production and increasing efficiency requirements leading to layoffs and redundancies as well as unemployment and unstable work careers which have, in turn, provoked various social problems in so-called vulnerable populations (for example, Charlesworth, 2000; Williams, 2003). The surge of global labour markets and the degradation of collective protection have led to the emergence of insecurity at the expense of a standard and stable employment relationship (Vosko, 2009; Benach et al, 2016). As an analytical concept, the use of the precariat and precarious work have gained popularity in this research realm. This idea places unequal forms of employment relations, economic and psychological insecurity, and the deterioration of career opportunities at the core of analysis.

Since the early 2000s this scientific approach to precarious work has highlighted the distinction between uncertain and unpredictable work contrasting with the relative security that characterized the three decades following the Second World War. One of the leading researchers of this area, Arne Kalleberg (2009), describes how the growth of precarious work since the 1970s has emerged as a major contemporary trend. According to this perspective, precarious work constitutes a global challenge that has a wide range of consequences, one of the key indicators being psychological and social suffering, associated with the fragile material wellbeing and poor future prospects. Therefore, it is considered important to analyse the new order of the economy that generates precarious work and worker insecurity, and on what scale precarious work generates mental vulnerability via uncertainty, unpredictability and material poverty (Tausig and Fenwick, 2011b).

Most literature on precarity suggests a direct connection between the characteristics of poor-quality jobs, unstable employment and the precarity of the subjects' lives. Indeed, it is a widely shared view that dependence upon precarious work has a negative impact on an individual's mental and physical health and wellbeing (Lewchuk et al, 2008; Kalleberg, 2011, 2018). This process begins with the character of jobs and employment, and finishes with the state of the individual (Barnes and Weller, 2020). At the core of this analysis are the declining employment relations that generate precarious work and the cultural and individual factors that impact people's responses to increasing uncertainty (Kalleberg, 2009). Researcher of labour market dynamics and precarity Guy Standing (2011, 2014) has proposed that the rise of unstable and insecure work has produced a growing social class – the 'precariat'. This analytical stand places the concern on precarious work as the determinant for precarious life. It stresses the absence of 'forms of labour-related security', which has set standards for decent employment in earlier labour market conditions, including opportunities to earn a monthly income, protection against arbitrary dismissal and a collective voice in the workplace (Kalleberg, 2011; see also Vosko, 2009).

To summarize, the precarity of work emphasizes how the development of the neoliberal market economy has impacted the security nets and negotiation power of employees, worsening their labour market status and leading to a new scale of work-related mental health problems. To avoid misunderstandings here it is highly important to note that in some definitions, precarious employment is limited to some disadvantaged 'precarious populations' but in more inclusive frameworks it refers to the 'processes of precarization', impacting adversely on larger proportions of employees and their employment/occupational/life conditions. It is therefore not a surprise that some researchers criticize the concept of precarious employment as being too fuzzy and containing a large variety of conceptualizations and operationalizations. This also leads to the fact that research on its actual impact on mental health indicators has been scarce (Rönnblad et al, 2019).

Although these approaches have raised important structural issues and macro-level transitions towards new forms of inequalities, they have remained rather silent on the historical changes of physical, institutional and cultural circumstances. For instance, in Finland chemical and physical hazards and harsh job conditions as well as poor living standards were typical characteristics of the post-war period of the 1950s and 1960s. High-speed urbanization caused numerous social and emotional problems, highly stigmatized ill mental health and poor availability of services made the use of adequate mental healthcare difficult, and occupational diseases and accidents were frequent. Although industrial and modern office jobs spread and living conditions improved in 1950–1970, many people lived in stressful conditions that some of today's researchers may label as precarious. Similarly, comparative supra-national studies provide a diverse perspective on the analysis of precarity. They show that different organizational and social political regimes facilitate or strengthen the precariousness of work while some other regimes can alleviate or cushion the amount and negative impacts of precarious work (Gallie, 2007; Clement et al, 2009; Campbell and Price, 2016; Kalleberg, 2018).

For these various reasons, it is important to reconsider what a position defined as a precariat looks like behind the statistics and in the thoughts of the subjects themselves (see also Gallie, 2007; Kalleberg, 2018). Grassroots level data and approaches may help to sharpen the analysis on the role of labour market transition in the formulation of mental vulnerabilities in relation to work and the lives of employees (McDovell et al, 2009), as well as how the position of work in life and the economic safety provided by the society are linked to precariousness and vulnerability.

From the socio-cultural perspective, I found research by Australian work sociologists Tom Barnes and Sally Weller (2020) interesting in terms of crafting precariousness and understanding the multidimensional nature of vulnerability. According to them, in Western societies, layoff involves multiple stages, from the announcement of job losses to the period of retrenchment, to the experience of job searching, to the acceptance of new jobs or withdrawal from the labour market. For workers laid off from long-term careers, their relations with states, markets and civil society therefore go through a process of transition. In terms of mental vulnerability, the structural (for example, social, political, material, cultural, organizational) contexts available provide an important framework for analysing the complex connections between unstable labour market, social norms of behaviour and mental vulnerability (see also McDovell et al, 2009; Anderson, 2010). According to Barnes and Weller it would be important to understand precarity through various economic, cultural and institutional mechanisms whereby risks are shifted, in multiple ways, from employers or state institutions onto individuals and households (Alberti et al, 2018). For instance, the protective mechanisms offered by societies differ sharply.

Weller and Barnes have studied the life trajectories and experiences of Australian blue-collar employees after being laid off. Their observations emphasize that it is the extent to which retrenched workers are already on a particular life trajectory at the time of their layoff that is what matters. Experienced employees are tied to the economic securities and benefits they have accrued (or been denied) through their long careers – that is, through their previous relations with markets, states and civil society. Instead of a uniform transition into precarity, researchers found a picture of diverse life trajectories:

> At one end of the spectrum, there was a relatively privileged group of workers who were shielded from market volatility and who could not be described as precarious in any meaningful way despite their exposure to insecure jobs. At the opposite end of the spectrum was a group of workers who were already in a precarious situation before the closure announcements. In between these two groups were the most retrenched workers, who had sufficient alternative income sources and a measure of asset wealth to provide short-term protection alongside ongoing exposure to precarious work. (Barnes and Weller, 2020)

The material on these manual workers from Australia has an interesting connection with our research materials from Finland. Our long-term research qualitative data on banking and insurance sector employees shows how redundancies and layoffs due to various organizational reorganizations were related to processes of 'precarization'. Economy-driven shifts had considerable social and emotional impacts for many employees who had been used to different labour market regimes and horizons of expectations (Varje, 2018; Kuokkanen et al, 2020). However, our materials also show how experiences and narratives have varied even within the same sector of employment. Crying industrial men burdened with layoffs or devalued female secretaries with excellent but outdated handwriting skills were only one part of the overall picture of labour market change between the 1960s and the beginning of 2000s when mental vulnerability became a societal problem in Finland (Wilkinson and Väänänen, 2021). Within a sector of decline or within the same organization under reorganization there were people who experienced harsh impacts of the market economy, but most people still moved towards the growing middle classes and their lifestyles. However, the burden caused by increasing organizational changes and speeding tempo were frequently mentioned in our interview materials as a source of increasing suffering (stress, burnout, exhaustion).

Norwegian social anthropologist Thomas Hylland Eriksen (2016: 114) has analysed these processes of globalization and free markets from the context of macro-level impacts on individual-level circumstances and life options. He characterized the situation of the 2010s as follows: 'Due to economic and technological changes, some people are not needed at the higher scale levels. Among the "trash" it is possible to find outdated know-how, substance abuse, and disadvantaged circles between generations in the context of rapidly changing labour market and requirements.' These external circumstances are reflected in psychological conditions that are experienced on the micro level. In this explanatory context, mental vulnerability is often linked to feelings of inferiority, lack of accomplishment, feelings of being in the wrong place and having to perform tasks that do not correspond to the ideals and norms of the social environment. The fundamental problem both in the understanding and treatment of mental health challenges is linked to biased interpretation of the scales. Problems are understood and intended to be managed at the individual level, but economic and social processes are more essential to understanding and managing an individual's situation. However, the examples from Finland and Australia indicate that the overly simplistic causal interpretations between macro structures and individual situations should be treated with caution (see also Kaplan, 2004). In other words, mental vulnerabilities manifested in national statistics, daily healthcare and work organizations are mediated by the historically changing aspects of social character. At the same time, how life difficulties (for example. problems in the labour market) arise as mental health issues vary according to the historical era and culture.

Based on both historical evidence and current European data sources (Eurostat, 2022), it seems justifiable to question the general hypothesis on the unified rise of precarious employment and particularly its impact on mental vulnerabilities in working-age populations. For instance, in Finland a nationally representative long-term analysis of work conditions revealed that the proportion of wage earners who worked in precarious jobs increased by only about 2 per cent between 1984 and 2013 (from 11 per cent 13 per cent) (Pyöriä and Ojala, 2016; see also Ojala et al, 2021). At the structural level, social benefits, opportunities for re-employment, a changing fit between the person and labour market, adult education, occupational rehabilitation system, and other components of social order offer changing settings to deal with labour market transitions. These dynamic conditions result in strategies to cope with difficulties and may help to reduce labour-market-related pressure on mental health-related activity (Bosmans et al, 2016). In addition, cultural practices and values of the historical era impact our opportunities to encounter the emerging threads as well as our ways to deal with dissatisfaction and agony related to precarious situations. For instance, according to our archival materials, unfair treatment in a workplace often resulted in interpersonal conflicts and small sabotages in the 1960s, while along the course of time it became more habitual to treat the inflamed situations with trained supervisors and/or psychologists or other health professionals. Along the social development, new frameworks of occupational wellness and mental wellbeing gained more space. The cultural and occupational transition of societies had a dramatic impact on how precarity was perceived, understood and coped with.

However, the analytical perspective of precarity seems to provide a relevant way for understanding the cruelty of contemporary work, and precarious position is often linked to trajectories of mental-health-related disability and drifting off from labour markets. However, the current volume and historical roots of the mental health crisis pinpoint a need for additional explanations for the surge of mental vulnerability. Bearing in mind the differences between countries in the volume of precarious work, for example in the EU (Mai, 2017), it seems likely that the considerable rise of mental vulnerability observed during the past 50 years is not likely to be explained by the large-scale rise of the precariat as a vulnerable class in Finland and other welfare societies alike. However, even though the precarious class may not be considerably expanding, it is important to analyse whether characteristics associated with precarious work have spread with an impact on the experiences of workers in a large variety of jobs. In this context, it is highly important to separate the discussion on the precarious class and nuanced dynamics of mental vulnerability and disability within the occupations and organizations. In the latter case, I think it is fairer and clearer to use other terms than precarious work or precarious life in welfare countries because mostly employees in permanent jobs have far more benefits and security than people who actually live their life in a precarious position.

4

The vulnerability of cultural existence

According to both the perspective of the deteriorating quality of work and the precarization of labour market, the rise in mental vulnerability has occurred because of exogenous changes related to economy and work. In contrast, critical research on population management has suggested that for the analysis of the late modern individual and labour market, rather than looking at the damaging effects of work on the person it is more important to examine the various practices that have been used to intervene in the subjectivity of employees. According to this view, the aim of a growing army of managers, researchers and experts has been the more efficient governing of persons at work and tackling the problems of human inefficiency more firmly (for example, boredom, overstrain, turnover, conflicts). This development of soft management, in turn, has had consequences related to the emergence of the psyche.

The critical approach of psychologization of work and health conceptualizes it from the perspective of individuals and social communities being consumed by potential narratives that stress psychological perspectives, therapeutic coping and genuine fulfilment of one's mental potential that might produce problems of vulnerability and erroneous conclusions that did not exist before (for example, Danziger, 1997; Furedi, 2004; Miller and Rose, 2008). This is seen as a potential factor that leads to disregarding structural problems, prioritizing a middle-class development-orientated worldview and/or ahistorical interpretations of work-related challenges that have developed during a long period of time.

In turn, the *second culturally critical* approach emphasizes the importance of medical discourses and medicine-related clinical practices and power structures in defining, framing and governing the challenges of work disability and mental wellbeing. This tradition points out how medicalization may influence the borders of mental normalcy and pathology in the domain of mental vulnerability (for example, Armstrong, 1995; Conrad, 2007; Horwitz, 2009). In this chapter, I will re-read and re-analyse specific issues that are regarded as important in each of these strands of scientific tradition in terms of how they can be used to explain mental vulnerability among the working-aged and in work organizations.

The shift towards psychological approaches

Analyses of psychologization of Western societies emphasize how academic psychology and/or psychological (from now on 'psy') conceptualizations, models of thinking and professional practices have started to occupy fundamental ideas of our thinking on the psyche in work and culture. In addition, they describe how various professionals have started to understand and define working conditions, social relations, group dynamics, organizational changes, individual differences, occupational hazards and other daily phenomena of work using psy-perspectives and languages.

In brief, the approach leads us to view the psyche as part of culture and knowledge-based exercise of power. It examines how psychologically alert approaches related to the vulnerable subjectivities are impacting today's work, working with the psyche and, ultimately, our own self-understanding. It also leads us to the question of whether we have such a different 'psychologized character' due to various societal changes that we now generate mental vulnerabilities that did not have a name or position some 50 or 60 years ago. Furthermore, are we so different so that it stimulates sensitivity to psychological issues and mental vulnerabilities (Furedi, 2004; McLaughlin, 2011)?

The analyses of psychologization have varied from the critical conceptual and etymological history of psychology (for example, Hacking, 1995; Danziger, 1997) to Foucauldian analyses of psy-cultures and psy-disciplines and of their ability to produce new adaptive self-regulating subjectivities (for example, Rose, 1996, 1999). The critical history of psychology and cognitive sciences reveals how psychological classifications and interpretations of human mentality have impacted our understanding of social behaviour and emotions (Danziger, 1997; Richards, 2002). Especially, during the 20th century, psychological thinking and profession secularized the soul and made it more approachable to the new population masses (Hacking, 1995). The institutional history of psychology, in turn, shows how professionals of psychology and the profession of psychology itself started to occupy a more important position in defining the work environment, work communities and employees as psychological subjects (Rose, 1996, 1999). However, it is essential to keep in mind the thought expressed by the philosopher of science Ian Hacking (1995: 40): 'A movement will "take" only if there is a larger social setting that will receive it.' So, to analyse the role of psychologization and its significance in the formation of mental vulnerabilities there is a need to understand how politicians, professionals, organizations and citizens started to call for and use a psychological understanding in work ability and mental wellbeing.

According to critical historian of psychology Graham Richards (2002) the appeal of psychological expertise originally lay in its promise that those possessing it would be able to more effectively manage the populations under their control. This 'management of individuality', as Nikolas Rose calls it, should not be mistaken for ruthless oppression, rather, according to Foucault-inspired interpretation, it took the form of extreme paternalism that seeks to steer employees and citizens in the desired direction by gentle means (Golder, 2007). In the early decades of the 20th century, psychological expertise had a considerable social demand as modernizing societies needed a better management of various social groups (for example, workers, soldiers, pupils) and their guidance towards self-managing and efficient citizenship. One of the main tasks of applied psychology was improving industrial productivity through a better understanding of phenomena such as mental fatigue and attention. It was this potential applicability of psychological expertise in war, in schools and at work that provided academic psychology's underlying cultural momentum and progressively gravitated it towards developing practical expertise (Newton, 1995; Rose, 1999; Richards, 2002).

According to the analyses of psychologization of Western cultures, the institutionalization of psychological knowledge in the population has led to a psychological understanding of occupational environments, personal capacities and social relationships but it has also impacted the essence of subjectivity. For instance, cultural sociologists Heidi Rimke and Jo Brock (2012) argue that struggling with one's psychological life has become a key cultural theme in modern life. According to them, especially North Americans seem to have a persistent impulse to worry about whether they are what they should be, and whether they have the sort of personal traits, skills, social manners or inner strengths they should have. In this context of psychological worry, experts translate various aspects of human life into myriad dysfunctions, addictions, disorders and pathologies and everyday psychological behaviours require special attention and self-treatment. The diversity of the psychological culture and the limitlessness of the psyche is what makes it so effective and self-growing: no one is ever really good enough.

In literature, a concept of therapeutic culture is often used to describe the psychological normalizing in culture (Nehring et al, 2020). It refers to cultural norms and values that invite individuals to constitute themselves as subjects who seek better self-knowledge and self-actualization (Salmenniemi, 2022). It also refers to a way of thinking and talking about ourselves and the world which uses psychological interpretations and categories of explanation and stresses the importance of adequate psycho-behavioural coping strategies. According to this view, we are dealing with a type of self-understanding and worldview which is historically recent and was popularized particularly during the 20th century (Gergen, 1991).

Norwegian cultural sociologist Ole Jacob Madsen (2018) has investigated the psychologization of Scandinavian societies. Among others he has investigated the major women's magazine *KK* in Norway. According to him, a conspicuous feature of *KK*'s lifestyle journalism is the therapeutic value of practically everything: physical activity ('Working out is like therapy for me'), attending cultural events ('Theatre is a cure for the mind and the heart'), hobbies ('She thought scrapbooking was like therapy'), pets ('Prescription of kittens'), gardening ('To plant seeds and watch them grow is better therapy than the best psychologist'), and so on. Although these articles in women's magazines can also be understood as a counterforce to the official culture of therapy, they nevertheless focus attention on the psychological wellbeing of the subject and emphasize the importance of revitalizing psychological processes through everyday behaviour.

Madsen (2018) has also studied the development of the therapeutic ethos in self-help literature and the discipline of psychology. Thanks to the growing influence of the self-help literature, concepts such as self-esteem, self-control, self-development and self-leadership have become the cornerstone of the current idea of a happy life. In Madsen's account, self-help literature is related to both the psychologization of everyday life and the development of psychological science. Psychology thrives on the public's insatiable thirst for self-knowledge. In turn, self-help literature typically uses and popularizes studies of psychology, cognitive science and related psy-disciplines (Madsen, 2018).

Two main strands of analyses can be distinguished in the analyses of psychologization: the analyses of 'public psychologization' deal with media, close relationships and self-help literature whereas the analysis of 'organizational psychologization' is a less studied area of psychologization. It focuses on the way work and organizational processes are psychologically managed, evaluated and led, as well as how employees are viewed, approached and supervised. Organization-based psychologization is also characterized by aspirations related to work ability and efficiency that are not so evident in the analysis of public psychologization focused more on psychological education, success narratives and therapeutic discourses. In this book, it is relevant to examine how psychological conceptualizations and practices contribute to the mental vulnerabilities we observe in different organizational contexts.

The work by Nikolas Rose (1989, 1996) on the progress of the psychological complex offers an important time window for the analysis of psychological knowledge in work. He has maintained that psychology's role should be understood from the historical needs and purposes of society and work. Rose has, for instance, analysed how the Second World War was crucial to psychology's full emergence as a discipline centrally concerned with what he calls 'technologies of subjectivity'. That is, concerned with devising technologies enabling the subjective realm to be rendered visible and quantifiable, in the form of graphs, scores, statistics and charts. Thanks to psychology, our intelligences can be measured, our personalities 'tested' and our mental distresses variously diagnosed as anxiety states, neuroses and stress disorders (Richards, 2002: 321, 330). In Rose's terms, our 'subjectivities' became 'inscribable and calculable'. Psychological knowledge has also been an important tool in improving employees' personal commitment and teamwork.

An illustrative example of the turn towards psychological capacities typically present in the labour market can be detected in job advertisements. In our research based on archival materials, we analysed job advertisements in the Finnish newspaper *Helsingin Sanomat*. It has been the largest newspaper in Finland since the 1920s and one of the most important national recruitment channels in Finland. It can be taken as a representative source of the trends in management and employee ideals. Our analysis of more than 2,000 advertisements revealed how the number and variety of skill requirements increased considerably between the 1950s and 2000s in the job advertisements. Especially expectations towards emotional and psychological skills increased and spread to various employment industries and job contents (Kuokkanen et al, 2013; Varje et al, 2013a, 2013b). The managerial advertisements reflected a considerable shift towards the anthropocentric management of subjectivities and the psychological climate (Varje et al, 2013a), while worker advertisements illustrated a drastic transition towards the psychological qualities of job seekers (Kuokkanen et al, 2013). In job advertisements employees were increasingly incited and instructed to be mentally adaptive and self-managerial as well as geared towards psychological development and psychological features of the job.

An important historical transition was seen between the late 1960s and the 1980s in terms of work, mental health and psychology. The quality of work and work stress paradigms emerged in several Western industrial countries (Väänänen et al, 2012). It can be viewed that since the 1970s, the new management-orientated work stress approach dealing with individuals' negative feelings and pressures at work reflected the basic shift in the occupational structure towards service and knowledge occupations and their work processes. As the proportion of heavy manual jobs declined, the role of 'psychological character' became increasingly important in several sectors of employment. It seems that the ideal of a production line worker who would perform routine tasks in a reliable way changed to become the ideal of a multi-skilled, emotionally capable team worker with good psychological adaptation (Varje et al, 2013a). This also entailed an increasing emphasis on the personal image and presentation of the self at the workplace (Adkins, 1995). The capacity for stress-fitness became a desired new employee characteristic in the last two decades of the 20th century (see also Newton, 1995). Through participatory work design, growing worker representation, job enrichment, self-managed work teams and so on, ideal work was viewed as more equal, satisfying and productive. One of the forerunners of this thinking was the Norwegian coalition project between various governmental parties and labour unions in the 1960s (Emery and

Thorsrud, 2013 [1969]). They focused on the development of industrial democracy and psychological meaningfulness of the job. These types of projects and many of their successors in other countries leant on social psychological expertise. For instance, formulations by social psychologists Kurt Lewin (1938) and Henry Murray (1938) that behaviour is built in interactive relation between the subject and the situation, provided a base for new psychology of work (Blau, 1981: 280–281) as well as new socio-cultural approaches of wellbeing at work (Hänninen, 1987). In the late 1900s, the ideals of organizational humanism were increasingly articulated in the name of stress reduction, personal fulfilment, the quality of the product, the efficiency of the enterprise and the political exemplariness of the company.

This line of thinking defined a company as an open system with its own psychological self-regulating properties and human actors. For instance, in the 1970s, the car manufacturer Volvo initiated a new mode of operation in Sweden where workers were granted more autonomy based on self-governing groups, and where new technology was used to facilitate the workers in their efforts, thus counteracting the tendency towards deskilling (for example, Womack et al, 1990). The socio-technical approach, psychological rationalization and humanization of work thereby favoured decentralization, which became a widespread strategy in the 1980s. According to Peter Miller and Nikolas Rose (2008: 186–190), these psychology-based projects provided organization managers with a new psychological way of acting upon their domain and gave them a social psychological vocabulary. However, in many countries the humanization of work and job redesign was rather marginal, and these ideas were absorbed into the managerial technology for promoting affective worker commitment. In the history of work and psychological thought, the period was characterized by the intentions to reform the quality of work through system-driven interventions. With the 'psychosocial' framework, a new image of the worker was also introduced by industrial and organizational psychology in the 1980s: a worker was more an individual seeking to fulfil him/herself through work. According to this view, work became an important path for a meaningful life. Psychological thinkers from Abraham Maslow to Victor Vroom crafted a new picture of the employee as an entrepreneurial individual seeking to psychologically fulfil him/herself in work and in all spheres of life (Rose, 1989; see also Väänänen et al, 2012).

Although differences and discontinuities existed in the labour market, the focus on the evolvement of individual and team-related psychological capacities spread in Western countries between the 1960s and 2000s. Psychological approaches and tools were often portrayed as potential sources of maintaining or recovering the capacity to work. A Swedish social anthropologist, Hans Tunestad (2014), has investigated management education, the healing of stress-related illnesses, the teachings of emotional intelligence in schools, and the representation of psychological tools in the mass media. According to him, they all follow the brainchild of self-help where the recipients are offered the possibility of becoming more able at work or simply becoming able to work once again. According to him, the change is connected to the structural transformation of contents and processes of work. While work has been therapeuticized, the ideal of strict organizational structures with a hierarchical control and command system has given way to that of smaller self-governing units organized in networks and mutual interdependences. As work here also takes on a more project-like character and entrepreneurial self-management is needed (Boltanski and Chiapello, 2007), this demands socio-emotional skills with co-workers who may be anything from full-time employees to 'temps' to consultants (see, for example, Furusten, 2003; Garsten, 2008).

The ideal social character in a work organization is no longer a toiler following orders from above, but a responsible and agentic individual (Meyer and Jepperson, 2000). Such a person is imagined to find the motivation inside the boundaries of work, such as the possibility for personal development and meaningful job contents, as well as mental wellbeing stimulated by work. The historical difference between eras could be described as follows: in the bureaucratic organizations and industrial plants of the early 20th century, psychological and social psychological techniques were used to increase profits and smoothen the contradictions between labourers and capital owners, whereas during the recent decades the evolvement of the psy-approaches have gained a more personal and individualistic character through the introduction of a reflexive and psychologically emancipatory worker. Listening to one's emotions, psychological self-care and authentic striving towards one' subjective life goals have become more significant in work as well as other areas of life.

The turn towards psychological knowledge, expertise and discourses in the labour market was linked to the development of non-hierarchical working cultures, the new demands of working processes and the overall focus on employee wellness. Even many stakeholders with strong advocacy positions such as labour unions adopted more acceptable views on psychological approaches and even therapeutic solutions in occupational health debates (McLaughlin, 2011). The improved management of psycho-emotional capacities and rationalization of psychological phenomena was required for several reasons. Critical organizational theorists have claimed that the orientation towards perspectives of organizational cultures and the psychologization of work (Bolton, 2005; Miller and Rose, 2008: 184; Fineman, 2010) coincided with a strong emphasis on harsh economic competition and neoliberal production of inequality (Harvey, 2005; Patomäki, 2007).

It is evident that the emphasis on more psychological forms of capital requiring innovations, customer satisfaction and flexibility led to the increased importance of psychological know-how. In this context, psychological dimensions became both culturally suitable and economically required. It can be interpreted that the growing emphasis on emotional wellbeing, employees' personal motivation and production of adequate feelings at work were signs of a new relationship between the psychoemotional employee and productivity. The strategic connection between emotional management and psychological knowledge in a changing economy suggests that if we want to understand psychologization we need to examine emotions and their changing role at work.

According to a synthesis of the organizational literature (Bolton, 2005: 14; Varje et al, 2013a) at least five distinctive processes related to the increased role of emotions in work organizations and work processes can be identified. At the cultural level, the emotionalization has been typically understood as the intensification of emotional discourse (for example, Holmes, 2010; Schmidt, 2021) and emotional subjectivity (for example, De Vos, 2013; Lerner and Rivkin-Fish, 2021). Different views on emotionalization offer essential ideas on how the processes of psychologization are related to the rise of mental vulnerabilities in work over the past decades in well-off Western countries. Next, I will briefly review the alternative interpretations for the *emotionalization* of work through which the rise of mental vulnerability can be viewed in the labour market.

The first approach focuses on the strategic role of emotions in production. It accepts the interpretation that the change towards emotional organizations has occurred through gradually developing practices of emotional management. For instance, Arlie Hochschild (1997) argues that organizations increasingly impose feeling rules for the employees, that is, emotional norms that they must follow. As an example, she analysed the work of flight attendants whose work is often characterized by emotional management and the importance of appropriateness of a feeling. According to these analyses, modern organizations choose which emotions they prefer and seek to restrain the expression of others (Wettergren and Sieben, 2010: 4). Pretentiousness and forced cheerfulness are examples of this in many professions in the service sector. According to this interpretation, the increasing focus on emotions reflects a transition from the control of external behaviour to a more refined form of management, which aims at more effective and less formal control of employees by attending to their thoughts and emotions (Burawoy, 1979; Barley and Kunda, 1992; Rose, 1999: 245–248). The psychology of emotional management provides tools for this. The proponents of labour process theory have viewed the psycho-emotional assimilation in organizations as a tool that increases the capitalist control over the work process (Braverman, 1974; see also Newton, 1995). From this perspective, work-related mental vulnerabilities could be seen as a potential outcome of increased emotional management of oneself and failed intentions to fulfil continuous requirements targeted towards appropriate emotions.

A second approach also utilizes the concept of increasing emotional control but offers a more materialistic and exogenous perspective. The economic growth in Western countries was exceptionally rapid during the period of 1950–1970. Alongside the educational expansion and growth in living standards, the late 1960s were characterized by popular reformist social movements, which targeted their criticism at areas such as the Tayloristic organization of work. Trade unionism was activated, the number of strikes increased significantly, and employers struggled with tense relations with employees (Haapala, 2006; Boltanski and Chiapello, 2007: 167–177; Julkunen, 2008: 102). However, during the 1970s, the strongest economic growth started to decelerate and the oil shocks caused economic difficulties (Boltanski and Chiapello, 2007: 184–194; Julkunen, 2008: 81–82). Organizations had to find the means to meet the demands of employees and to increase their productivity. In this historical context, the development of personnel management and de-bureaucratization of organizational structures emotionalized the work environment (Cascio, 1995; Smith and Thompson, 1998; Clausen and Olsen, 2000; Ezzy, 2001; Julkunen, 2008: 120–146). According to many critical views, by the 1980s attention to individual needs, emotional assimilation and wellness discourse had replaced the collectivism and activism of the 1960s and 1970s in the labour market (Clausen and Olsen, 2000; Wainwright and Calnan, 2002: 126; Boltanski and Chiapello, 2007; Siltala, 2007).

The economic-political change during the 1970s and 1980s has been interpreted as a break between the old Tayloristic organization and the new flexible organization. As was described in the earlier chapter of this book, the slowdown of economic growth and deregulation of national economies increased competitiveness in business and labour markets, and organizational reforms towards greater flexibility became important tools for improved efficiency (de Wolff, 1994; Boltanski and Chiapello, 2007: 195; Siltala, 2007; Julkunen, 2008: 103–107). Psychological understanding was increasingly needed in this demanding situation. This also signified a greater attention to human resources and psychological features of work. Motivation and commitment became important assets and increasing pressure towards management of 'psychosocial' and 'wellbeing' spread in work organizations.

The approaches described here share the view that the new models of management consider feelings and creativity as potential ways in which to increase productivity and efficiency. In this context, the display and management of emotions is acknowledged as rational business behaviour (Hughes, 2005; Boltanski and Chiapello, 2007: 98; Baumeler, 2010: 280; Imdorf, 2010: 94). In this way, more efficient methods for organizing the psychological management of employees seemed like a potential way of increasing productivity via increasing psychological capital.

However, a third approach describes the emotionalization of work in terms of increasing equality and liberalization of emotions. A Dutch sociologist, Cas Wouters (2007), argues that the increasing social complexity and democratization of Western societies has resulted in an informalization process that has reduced the formal control of emotions and increased the need for emotional sensitivity in social interaction. Indicatively, among the demands of the critics of Tayloristic work from the 1960s onwards were emotional rewards, interpersonal contacts, equality and sensitivity to differences (Boltanski and Chiapello, 2007: 97). The social reformist movement also included ideologies that promoted leadership styles considered feminine, including psychologically attentive behavioural styles such as listening and interaction (Pedriana, 2004). From the point of view of cultural liberalisation, it seems obvious that transition in social codes and behavioural structures has increased the need for psychological know-how and opened a cultural space for the emergence of new mental vulnerabilities.

A fourth, most materialistic and often overlooked approach is to view the change in organizations from the perspective of work content, organization and technology. From the 18th century to the present, industrialization has been characterized by the increasing mechanization of production, which originally caused more and more low-skilled workers to be tied to the repetitive pace of the machines. However, especially from the late 1960s onwards, increasing automatization has reduced the proportion of routine physical tasks, causing the workforce to be transferred to more information management and human interaction (Autor et al, 2003; Spitz-Oener, 2006). Not only has the proportion of employees in service and knowledge sectors increased and the proportion of employees in manufacturing decreased, but also in manufacturing the proportion of employees in psychologically demanding jobs increased (Berman et al, 1994). Work that demands networking and reading emotions has not only spread to new trades and occupations but also general strategies to cope with emotional and social challenges among working populations have edged towards the psychological management. These changes have been accompanied by organizational reformations towards reduced external control and increased teamwork, again creating a more emotionally orientated work environment (Kira, 2003: 62; Olsen, 2006). An example of this could be, for example, the popularity of the concept of psychological safety which has been raised alongside the traditional occupational safety. A work community with emotional openness and permissiveness plays an important role in it.

Fifth, a moral behaviour-orientated reinterpretation of the psychologization of the late modern employee has been offered by social historian of psychology Peter van Drunen and colleagues (2003). According to them, what Max Weber once called the 'protestant ethic' has now been replaced by a 'psychological ethic' (van Drunen et al, 2003: 161). In earlier periods of Protestantism, the contract with eternal life was dependent on decency and the diligence of work you had managed to deliver to serve God. In the new cultural constellation, the contract was made with the modern organization. In this new contract, emotional involvement, satisfaction and meaningfulness produced by work were the essential parts of this relationship. The basic meaning of work moved from the spiritual and religious arena to an emotional and psychological arena filled with me-related objectives and individualistic values.

On a macro-sociological level, this line of argument includes the idea of a considerable historical transition in the motivational structure of working agency. Whereas Weber (1978) described a situation where economic rationality was an effect, a sort of by-product, of a spiritual conviction, the 'spiritual' dimension is here consciously introduced as a way of accomplishing a more efficient work process. Managing by making use of psychological tools, thus attempting to instil a psychological work ethic as well as emotions and how to lead and fulfil them are key aspects of new 'spiritual economy' (Rudnyckyj, 2009).

Taken together, critical analyses provide important insights for capturing the rise of the psychology-orientated character in the work and labour market. This transformation has been manifested in the new concepts such as 'mental', 'psychological' and 'emotional' capital (Goleman, 1996; Luthans, 2007; Cooper et al, 2010) that became popular in both scientific and quasi-scientific discussions in the late 1990s and early 2000s (Weiskopf and Munro, 2012; Tunestad, 2014). By linking individuals, groups and organizations, psychological approaches make the enterprise culture appear less as a way of stressing the 'individual' on behalf of the 'social' and more as an alternative way of configuring these two (Collier, 2011; Tunestad, 2014). By indicating the psychosocial benefits of efficient work – that is, how work and wellbeing underpin each other – management-driven psychology repeatedly argues that psychologically successful work benefits everyone and thus that is in the service of the common good (cf Boltanski and Chiapello, 2007: 16). In this manner, the psychologization of society is typically seen as a negative process in critical literature in which political, moral and social issues have been reduced to a matter of psychological factors, thanks to psychology's growing entanglement with neoliberal forms of governance (see also Madsen, 2018).

Although these analyses provide us with conceptual tools for developing alternative pathways for understanding of mental vulnerability at work, their analytical perspective is somewhat limited. For instance, these interpretations can be criticized for drafting a manipulative figure of an employee who is exposed to the micro-power derived from psychological governing most evident in therapeutic discourses and management procedures. The used empirical material might partly affect this interpretation. Self-help literature, women's magazines and psychology-driven texts are typical sources of information in the analysis of therapeutization or psychologization of culture (Danziger, 1997; Furedi, 2004; De Vos, 2013; Madsen, 2021). Similarly, management guidebooks, learning materials and policy reports are typical materials of critical organizational studies analysing psychologization and its negative side-effects (for example, Rose, 1999; McLaughlin, 2012; Mannevuo, 2020). These types of non-worker-related materials are often presented as essential sources of information regarding psychologization. Within this analytical framework, the shop-floor level of occupational health and the history of organizational wellbeing have often remained superficially explored topics and scarce data exists on how long-term transitions in the psychologization of occupational life have changed the position of mental vulnerability in the labour market.

The view on the passive subjectivity of psychological toolbox users does not correspond to the results of organizational analyses stressing the importance of active relational agency in the formulation of workership and wellbeing (Olakivi, 2018; Newton et al, 2022). For instance, employees representing different organizational positions or industries are likely to have quite different views on the importance of psychological understanding for their identity. The 'toolbox' is not automatically contaminated by psychological concepts and thought structures. Hence, rather than viewing the relationship between neoliberalism and psychologization/therapeutization as necessarily co-terminous and mutually supportive, it is more analytical to view the gradual development of psychological approaches and therapeutic culture as ambiguous and historically shifting (Salmenniemi, 2022: 13). The current surge of mental vulnerability calls for a detailed analysis of the use of psychological approaches in the formation of mental vulnerability in different locations of the labour market and health services.

It is also noteworthy that many critical studies on the transition of work and workers towards psychological models of thinking are rather descriptive and theoretical in nature. These approaches have also paid little attention to collective processes impacting historical subjectivity of employees such as the development of labour unions, the socio-cultural change of the labour force, and the social class transition during a long time span. For instance, in Finland, the 'psy-education' of the workforce was influenced by various state-run political programmes and governmental interventions (for example, introduction of occupational health legislation and psychological safety regulations). The change of occupations and organizations created a need for psychological knowledge. As new generations entered work, the contents of work change, and ways of management became more civilized, psychological wellbeing and ill-being at work became topics of discussion.

The quest for historical and local subjectivity also leads to several important questions: How may psychological language have changed the official management of work and work ability? How do subjects who are 'governed' or 'classified' or 'psychologized' understand and conceptualize their situation? How have their behavioural registers and emotional landscapes changed during the period of psychologization? How are fundamental changes in work contents and processes related to their psychologization among employees and professionals? How has the ideal social character changed as psychological understanding and emphasis have stepped in? How might the alleged change be reflected in employees' behaviour in occupational health? I will discuss these topics in later chapters, in which the results of our own studies are presented in more detail. Before moving on to these themes, there is a need to discuss the sibling of psychologization, medicalization.

Medicalization and mental health at work

In the *Finnish Journal of Social Medicine*, social psychiatrist Sami Pirkola (2019) commented that a new discussion on mental health had been initiated over the past years. According to him, there had been more discussion on loneliness among older people, poor mental wellbeing among younger people, anxiety related to climate change, and difficulties in getting in psychotherapy treatment. Social historian Anna Kinnunen (2020b: 97) interprets that these sort of heterogeneous examples indicate the broadening of scope of mental health in current Western society. Mental health covers various symptoms, behaviour and illness. This blurring and spreading of the boundaries of mental health is observable in the population health statistics. When we compare the current status of mental health with the historical data, we are able to observe a considerable change. In 1940 about 1 per cent of the Finnish population was estimated to suffer from mental disorders (Kaila, 1942), whereas in the early 2000s the corresponding percentage was estimated to be around 20 per cent (Joukamaa, 2002: 286). Correspondently, international reports have reported a higher prevalence of mental-health-related disabilities after the 2000s than ever before (Wittchen and Jacobi, 2005; Abate et al, 2018).

Sociological studies of the 'medicalization of life' provides valuable insights concerning the institutional and cultural widening of mental health illnesses (Szasz, 1961; Conrad, 2007). According to the well-known researcher of medicalization Peter Conrad (2007), medicalization is a process by which non-medical problems become defined and treated as medical problems, usually in terms of illness and disorders (2007: 4). The key to medicalization therefore is the definition: a problem which is 'defined in medical terms, described using a medical language, understood through the adoption of a medical framework, or "treated" with a medical intervention' (2007: 5). To 'medicalize' something then, in short, is quite literally 'to make medical' (Conrad, 2007: 5; Bröer and Besseling, 2017).

The approaches focusing on medicalization emphasize the development of medical expertise and the strengthening role of medical institutions in defining and managing the issue of work ability and health. The analyses often stress increasing identification of risk factors, redefining the boundary between normal and pathological, and expanding psychiatric diagnostics, as well as the transfer of various everyday experiences to the arena of medical management (for example, Shorter, 1997; Conrad, 2007; Helén, 2007a; Miller and Rose, 2008; Petersen and Wilkinson, 2008; Kincaid and Sullivan, 2014; Väänänen et al, 2019).

According to several medical historians and social scientists (for example, Horwitz, 2003; Helén, 2010; Brinkmann, 2016), the drastic transition in mental health was influenced by an epidemiological transition in psychiatry around the 1950s and early 1960s. The American Psychiatric Association developed a new version of the diagnostic and statistical manual of mental disorders (DSM) and the World Health Organization launched an international classification on diseases (ICD) which classified and finally defined psychiatric disorders according to symptoms and not according to social circumstances or epidemiological factors. The simplest way of illustrating the medicalization of mental health is perhaps the growth of the number of pages in the DSM manual: the original DSM-I (1952) was 130 pages long, listing 106 disorders. By its fourth edition, published in 1994, DSM-IV was 886 pages long and listed 297 disorders, thus nearly triple the number (Grob, 1991; Rimke and Brock, 2012). The controversial DSM-V in 2013 reached a length of 947 pages by including new mental disorders and several subcategories for older disorders.

It is justly argued that cultural pathologies, as well as the language and discourses related to mental health problems, became better known as our culture became more diagnosis-oriented (Brinkmann, 2016). At the same time, short tests related to anxiety and depression became popular in media. This transition has led to a situation in which various kinds of behaviours, emotions and changes in functional ability are associated with mental disorders and interpreted from the psychiatric perspective (Busfield, 2000; Helén, 2010; Karp, 2017). Studies on medicalization propose that medical categorizations and the treatment practices related to mental health problems fuel the spread of medical worldviews and categories associated with low mood, personal problems and other social and emotional challenges in life (for example, Horwitz, 2003).

The traditional studies of medicalization have often stressed the unwanted and even damaging effects of medicalization (Goffman, 1961; Scheff, 1967). They have been based on top-down models that emphasize the status and role of mental health professionals and researchers in the emergence of the phenomenon (Bröer and Besseling, 2017). These analyses have often highlighted the disabling and disenfranchising role of medicalization for patients in the treatment of mental health problems (Broom and Woodward, 1996). However, more recent studies on the dynamics of demedicalization versus medicalization (Halfmann, 2012), patients' activity (Broom, 2005) and the social spreading of medical labels (Liu et al, 2010) have challenged the top-down models of medicalization. They suggest a multidimensionality, which also includes the tendency to challenge medical power when defining and framing mental health problems.

Given these historical transitions, it is important to distinguish the process of medicalization from the concept of medical dominance. Medical dominance is part of medicalization and refers to the power of doctors to determine policy decisions (Broom and Woodward, 1996). As the medicalization of mental health problems and the estimation of their seriousness with psychological and psychiatric instruments (for example, Beck Depression Inventory, Maslach Burnout Inventory) has spread, the medical dominance of doctors has been scrutinized and has even become controversial over the last decades. In fact, the deterioration of traditional medical dominance has been fuelled by both cultural changes in patient cohorts (Brown et al, 2015) and changes in the models of interaction promoted among doctors (Charles et al, 1999).

However, surprisingly little research on medicalization among employees has focused on the historically unique social arenas in which the actual definitions and categorizations concerning the medical status of employees' mental health take place. For the social research of mental vulnerability at work, it would be essential to analyse how the rules and norms that define the normal and pathological are constructed and negotiated, how everyday medical encounters defining the position of the psyche have changed and how changes in the interface between employees and doctors resonate with changes in the labour market (see also Durkheim, 1964). In line with this, historians of psychiatry emphasize that changing socio-cultural norms concerning mental wellbeing, as well as favoured behavioural models, deeply influence the way in which mental health concerns have been conceptualized, expressed and acted out (for example, Shorter, 1997). For instance, favoured human characteristics, like being active versus passive, solution-seeking versus resigned, open versus reserved, psychologically fit versus physically robust, have gained meaning in the historical setting, and this is something which is likely to be manifested in the descriptions of symptoms, adopting the sick role, and in thresholds and reasons for visiting a doctor (for example, Väänänen et al, 2019).

It is reasonable to argue that treating mental activity in a medical context and structuring it from the mental health framework positions psychological vulnerability in the medical realm while altering the employee's role as a patient. Related to the drastic transitions in work and the societal landscape (for example, educational level, efficiency requirements, psychological approaches), the handling of emotional distress and disability issues has undergone dramatic change. For instance, medical dominance has no longer been so present in consultations in the 2010s and 2020s and doctors are more willing to enter into reciprocal interaction with their patients (Broom and Woodward, 1996). Studies indeed propose that the patients' involvement in the medical encounter (Renedo et al, 2018) is increasing, and that the idea of doctors acting in partnership with patients is growing (Elston, 2009; Väänänen et al, 2019). In addition, it seems that in many cases, the reflexivity of patients has been augmented, and they also need to have their experience 'constructively medicalized' (Broom and Woodward, 1996). Indeed, the rise in the status of mental health has taken place at the same time as earlier asymmetries between doctors and patients have been challenged and the codes of formal interaction have lost their power (McKinlay and Marceau, 2002). However, little is known about how the changes have affected the work of medical professionals with working people, or how the increasing prevalence of a potentially more reflexive social character and awareness of psychiatric categories may have been associated with the rise of mental vulnerability over the last decades.

The descriptions of patient encounters can provide important information on the intertwined reasons for patients' health complaints and the medical practices that define mental health problems. In one of our interview studies, we gathered material on the accounts of senior medical professionals (mainly senior occupational health doctors) who had worked in occupational healthcare from the late 1960s to the early 2010s on how they have viewed the changing employee populations in relation to mental health, how they interpreted the changing role of mental health at work, and how they have experienced changes in the diagnostic culture (Väänänen et al, 2019). These physicians' accounts can be seen to indicate the link between the historicity of employee mental health and the medicalization process, as well as reflect the normalization of the contemporary mental pathologies among employees (for example, Busfield, 2000, 2011; McLaughlin, 2011; Wainwright and Calnan, 2011; Brinkmann, 2016).

According to our interviews, in the 1960s and 1970s, the concept of mental ill-health mainly referred to mental disorders such as neuroses and severe diseases such as schizophrenia. Mental problems were strongly associated with pathology and lunacy. The psychological and social challenges often described by today's employees were rare in occupational health care at the time. If a physician made a diagnosis of depression, the common answer was 'I am not a maniac'. The images that the interviewees offered of the period up to the late 1980s thus emphasized the reluctance of employees to discuss mental health problems and the psychological stresses of work with a doctor. The way in which the interviewees represented the gradual cultural change was often illustrated with the observation of how employees started to view themselves and act differently. Employees gradually began to perceive knowledge seeking and expertise within the medical realm as a potential solution when faced with mentally strenuous circumstances or problems. Within this new behavioural constellation, medical services were increasingly used for purposes of personal coping.

The interviewees felt that the medical basis of many diagnoses was not always clear in the new active culture of care brought by new clients that took actively care of their mind, and that the diagnostic labels could not be evaluated within a biomedical framework alone. For instance, job burnout was often viewed as a problematic diagnosis because it did not ensure the patient the same sickness benefits as depression in the Finnish imbursement system. This suggests that new behavioural challenges became part of the medicalization process and doctors had controversial feelings about them. The growing categories of mental health diagnoses were influenced by factors outside the system of disorder categories, such as the evaluation of social benefits (Järvensivu et al, 2018). The problems, in turn, reflected the broader change in production and culture (cf Williams et al, 2008).

Our analysis suggests that the re-positioning of the social stigma related to mental health was strongly related to the transition of the social and occupational frameworks among Finnish employees. In the interviews, the older physicians directly stressed the importance of transition in the social character. In the 1970s, many patients had experienced war. Daily life had been materially challenging for many. The doctors emphasized that it was simply not an option for employees to seek professional help for a mentally difficult situation. It was about knowledge, but also about ways of doing things that were considered natural. Physicians were considered to be at the top of the occupational hierarchy, and they felt their relations with their patients through their hierarchical status. In the 1960s and 1970s, physically, biologically and chemically hazardous working conditions needed various improvements. Concerns related to employees' moods or psychological problems did not easily land on the physician's plate. However, the interviewees argued that there was a gradual shift in the social criteria of structuring and perceiving psycho-emotional states in the working-aged population between the 1970s and 2000s (Väänänen et al, 2019).

Several interviewees argued that the growth of mental challenges was associated with a diminished ability to cope with daily worries and obstacles at work. Especially many older doctors relate this 'modernity syndrome' directly to a change in the social character of the employees. This is manifested in comments such as "the old type of guts has disappeared". Doctors saw a sharp contrast with their own personal past. For instance, the sorrow related to a pet's death was dealt with without the help of healthcare professionals in the 1970s and 1980s. The situation was different in the 2010s.

Numerous doctors claimed that society's public safety norms and caring institutions have overdeveloped and gone too far. Their own autobiographical perspective led them to suspect patients' intrapersonal resiliency when faced with psychological pain and challenges in life.

At the same time, the context within which the doctors interpreted the changing behaviour of the patient represented not only a cultural shift, but also a macro-level transition in the economy and the population. Still in the 1950s, primary and secondary production together represented about 70 per cent of the employment share, but by 2000 more than 60 per cent of Finnish employees worked in the service sector (Hannikainen and Heikkinen, 2006). After the 1980s, the information society and its related occupations and contents of work spread. Many traditional jobs consisting of physical tasks were eliminated, and the new jobs increasingly required digital skills and mental and cognitive capacities (Varje, 2018). In addition, the educational level of the Finnish workforce rose rapidly (Statistics Finland, 2010). New market economy started to assign prestige to different social and mental characteristics among employees as part of productivity (Kuokkanen et al, 2013). These structural processes were reflected in physicians' work with employees who found it increasingly difficult to cope with the demands of the new work culture.

> 'The changing society is strongly involved. ... Job opportunities just appeared (in the late 1960s and 1970s), baby boomers were pushed into the labour market and industry was developing. Companies educated their staff. When these people were in their 40s in the 1990s, they were completely uneducated, they had nothing. Or they had some type of competency, but not what was needed. There was Nokia and the high-tech boom, but they were not suitable then.' (Male doctor, born in 1942, started practising in the 1960s)

According to their views, the structural transitions in the economy and society contributed to a considerable shift towards the management of psychological suffering in everyday life. Doctors utilized many sociological interpretative frameworks, as they viewed the growth of mental health concerns from the perspective of the macro-level transition in production and the socio-cultural characteristics of the population (Moloney, 2017). They referred to the transition of work, organizational changes, devaluation of traditional skills, medicalization of everyday problems, the transition of generations, the loosening of mental health stigma, and so on, but they hardly ever refer to the transition of the biological or physiological environment or the corporeal basis of their patient. This is a very critical and social perspective towards medicalization compared to earlier research about the medicalization of classification systems. However, it is also the case that the medical industry transformed the challenges of everyday life, such as attention deficit disorders or symptoms of anxiety, into a medical challenge, and this increased the diagnostic arsenal of scientific psychiatry, which in turn also reached informed employees and their doctors.

There is no doubt that occupational health physicians and other occupational health professionals had to adapt themselves to the changing circumstances. The change of the whole labour market and the cultural developments, and new behavioural forms and challenges of the population, were something doctors were forced to reflect and act upon when addressing psycho-emotional challenges that were increasingly perceived as mental health problems. These developments were conceived to be neither good nor bad, but as having a rather paradoxical character. Many doctors felt quite helpless in the face of these advancements, even though they recognized that the earlier silence on the topic was not good either. These problems were often something that inhabited the liminal space between pathology and normalcy (Gabe and Bury, 1988; Moloney, 2017). These types of findings shed more light on the intersection between changing society, work and mental health in processing mental vulnerabilities by exploring the different ways in which the transforming employee requirements and developing social norms of psychosocial life were reflected in mental problems faced by employees, daily coping strategies, diagnostic categorizations, and the overall value judgements of mental health problems (for example, Totton, 2006; Brinkmann, 2016). From this point of view, medicalisation is positioned at the interfaces of a changing society and work culture, where historical agency is transformed and takes on new kinds of manifestations. The shift towards dealing with subjective states and becoming an employee who relies on mental work ability thus also meant the emergence of personal experience and new mental health in occupational health care.

A simplistic argument states that the spreading of therapeutic cultural codes and medicalization of mental health among younger generations has caused the emergence of mental vulnerability. However, the evident link with the macro-economy and personal vulnerabilities calls for a more systematic analysis that combines cultural-level explanations (for example, psychologization, medicalization) with an analytical framework that considers changes in the production and economy. For example, this means changing employee ideals and ability requirements at work as part of the formation of vulnerability. All in all, the historical analysis of medicalization of mental health in the context of work provides an important time window for understanding the surge of mental vulnerability in the context of a changing society. It indicates how various simultaneous processes such as the population's increased level of psycho-emotional mobilization and the transition of occupational structure as well as the expansion of medical knowledge towards social areas of life contributed to the gradual emergence of mental health concerns as we know them in the 2020s.

Also findings from both cross-cultural psychology (Shiraev and Levy, 2020) and comparative social research (for example, Arikan and Bloom, 2015) indicate that Western assumptions about work-related mental health and understanding of adequate expressions of mental uneasiness are non-universal. Problems with ethnocentrism and ahistorical understanding can be seen as concrete research challenges. Within current cultural context, risk-aware Western employees probably observe, interpret, narrate and counteract more upon psycho-emotional 'exposures' and 'stressors' in their social relationships. Overall, if we accept that mental vulnerability is a historically and culturally specific phenomenon, we need to look at the historical circumstances in which the needs for new behavioural strategies and forms of mental vulnerability have evolved. It is time to move on to the study of the historical emergence of mentally problematic subjectivities in modernizing societies.

5

Mental vulnerability in the historical context

The explanatory frameworks of the social sciences typically analyse the current situation concerning mental vulnerability and the impact of recent societal and organizational change. Since over a long period of time, views on the challenges of the psyche and their treatment have changed, historical studies of mental health and social behaviour can open an essential perspective for today's understanding on mental vulnerability. In this chapter, I will present a history-driven approach on how mental vulnerabilities have emerged as a part of the transition of societal conditions impacting human existence.

To contextualize our current situation, I will first review some evidence concerning the historical changes in the understanding of mental vulnerabilities. Then I will discuss the models of epidemiological transition to show how normalized understanding in health and population sciences views long-term changes in population health. In the last part, I shall examine a late modern subject that has received little attention in epidemiological and historical examination and consider a new structure of social behaviour as a generator of mental vulnerability and need for managing the human mind.

Mental vulnerabilities of the past

The rise of mental vulnerabilities has been viewed in sociological terms as an effect of a society marked by restrained competition, inequality, medicalization and psychologization. History-focused contributors focusing on the formation and conceptualizations of mental vulnerabilities, in turn, adopt a perspective based on the history of culture, behaviour, ideas and institutions. The analysis of present manifestations of mental vulnerability can be viewed as part of the historical trajectory of concepts and the normative history of social life among humans (Neckel et al, 2017). In this way, historical research of mental health provides important insights into wellbeing at work and the temporal flavour of mental health problems (Pietikäinen, 2013).

According to a social history of mental health, the first documented discussions on mental difficulties and exhaustion took place in the era of the humoral tradition. The Greek physician Galen of Pergamon (129–216 CE) suggested that there was no clear distinction between the body and the soul, between the mental and the physical. He hypothesized that 'passions' caused mental health problems and the disorganization of the whole body. In line with the humoral tradition, he suggested that mental health was based on four bodily humors: blood, yellow bile, black bile and phlegm. In Galen's writings, lack of mental energy was presented as a core concern and it manifested in the guise of lethargy, torpor, weariness and sluggishness (Schaffner, 2017: 29). The cure for this kind of symptomology entailed blood-letting, but he also suggested a sort of mental health counselling that has similarities with current psychotherapies. Among others, it included a confession of deepest passions and secrets to an older and wiser man who himself was free from passions (King, 2009).

One of the most important concepts of mental health that became popular in the sciences and theology of the early modern times was named acedia (or 'sloth'). This was first described by the monk and theologian Evagrius Ponticus (346–399 CE). Its symptoms included sleeplessness, irritability and hopelessness, but also impatience and agitation which were manifested in various unproductive displacement activities according to Pontius. During the next centuries, acedia had a considerable role in the theological texts and many different definitions were developed. Often theological worldviews considerably impacted the etiological understanding on the roots of acedia. From today's perspective, it could be seen as an exhaustion of early modernity caused by sinful behaviour. In the Middle Ages, an influential Italian philosopher and priest Thomas Aquinas (1225–1274) labelled acedia as a form of spiritual apathy manifested in the rejection of the effort required to commit oneself to God (Schaffner, 2017: 35–36). The state often referred to 'a cessation of motion and an indifference to work' that manifests itself as inactivity and was often interpreted as laziness (Lyman, 1989: 5; Issakainen, 2016: 55).

The early texts on exhaustion and depression provide examples of the ways problems related to mental fragility and management were seen before our historical period, which is characterized by biomedicine, applied psychology and secularized society. The Christian framework linking sins and mental suffering maintained its role in the attributions describing the sources of mental illness and debility until the later period of scientific revolution in the 18th century. Within these frameworks of thinking, mental suffering and psychological problems were typically understood in corporeal and theological terms. Philosophers, theologians and ancestors of modern medicine were important developers of knowledge, dominating the topic of mental vulnerability before the advent of modern biomedicine and psychiatry. The early history of mental health problems shows how problems with the psyche and their interpretations were heavily influenced by temporal ideals and moral values concerning the constitution of the body and correct behaviour leading to a 'good life'. These traditions were also important for suffering people and their families for centuries as humoral theory, for instance, remained the dominant medical paradigm until the advent of modern medicine in the 19th century.

Since the era of Enlightenment, scientific theories gained more popularity and began to claim that human nature was the result of biological, physiological and/or psychological factors. Gradually Western theories shifted towards scientific rather than theological explanations. Positivists insisted that through systematic observation, human behaviour could be explained in the same objective manner as the hard sciences explained the natural world. Critical social historians have argued that scientific and quasi-scientific discourses and practices that emerged from the Enlightenment onwards had a profound effect on how people and their pathologies were understood, and how people themselves also changed (for example, Foucault, 2003, 2005).

By the mid-to-late-19th century, the human sciences developed numerous new branches of study, such as phrenology, anthropology, neurology, craniology, criminology, experimental psychology, physiognomy, necrology and psychological medicine (Rimke and Brock, 2012). The new science of the soul, psychiatry, claimed that madness, melancholy or other mental health problems were not the result of demonic possession or a punishment from God or animatic passions, but disease entities that required medical attention. Although religious worldviews, humoral theories and old paradigms of the human body still impacted both lay and professional views on mental health and ill-health in the 19th century (Laqueur, 1992; Porter, 1997), the formation of a medical model of mental pathology was gradually developed and overcame earlier explanations. At the same time, the scientific search for endogenous causes rooted in the human body became a hallmark of modernity (Rimke, 2008; Rimke and Brock, 2012).

As a form of modernized acedia, an American neurologist, Georg M. Beard, developed a detailed description of the symptomatology and pathology of neurasthenia in the 1870s. Although he worked outside academia as an electro therapist and neurologist with this far-reaching conceptualization, he soon gained wide popularity with books such as *American Nervousness* (Beard, 2008 [1881]). In his research, he located the illness primarily in members of the new urban middle and upper classes of the north and east United States, in so-called brain workers: businessmen, lawyers, scientists, engineers, journalists, politicians, doctors and clergymen (Kury, 2017: 54). He suggested that it was the living conditions of the technologized modern age with its new modes of transport, communication, mass media and technologies that put the human nervous system under greater strain than in the past (see Schnittker, 2021: 15–21).

'Neurasthenia was the signature disease of the time', social historian Anna Schaffner (2017) states. It was regarded as a consequence of urbanization, industrialization and technological progress, thus, key processes of modernization. The living and working conditions of bourgeois elites had been transformed in a short time by technological innovations. In the public understanding these societal changes were thought to lead to symptoms such as irritability, exhaustion and insomnia. Abuse of drugs was also characteristic of the era, according to Beard. The idea of exogenous suffering was embodied in the character of the new 'societal disease': external conditions were reflected in internal psychological states (for example, Neckel et al, 2017: 6). Beard defined neurasthenia as a clinical syndrome, as a disease of civilization, related to the modern lifestyle with its achievement orientation (Kury, 2017: 55–59). The neurasthenia framework and its various interpretations spread widely in the early 1880s and reached its heyday before 1900 (Kury, 2017: 55). In the 1880s and 1890s, upper social class people of many central European areas (Germany and Austria in particular) thought they were living in an age of exhaustion (Neckel et al, 2017).

From the historical context of rising urbanization and the stimulation of new lifestyles, it seems natural that physicians and scientists noted the transition and attributed the rise of mental health problems to overactivation, speed and the hectic rhythm of modern life. From this perspective, it is not only a coincidence that the period of modernization in the West signified the birth of modern social sciences, including sociology, social psychology and social anthropology, which have often analysed the social impacts of modernization on human communities and mental wellbeing.

A sociologist of modernization, Georg Simmel, described the fundamental problem in *The Metropolis and Mental Life* (1950 [1903]) as follows:

> The psychological basis of the metropolitan type of individuality consists of the intensification of nervous stimulation which results from the swift and uninterrupted change of outer and inner stimuli. … Intellectuality is thus seen to preserve subjective life against the overwhelming power of metropolitan life. … Punctuality, calculability, exactness are forced upon life by the complexity and extension of metropolitan existence and are not only most intimately connected with its money economy and intellectualist character. (Simmel, 1950 [1903]: 13)

Another German sociologist of the same period, Max Weber, in turn, considered the modern society as an iron cage, stressing the importance of pressures on an individual's emotional experience organized by Western rationalism and capitalism. He emphasized the role of culturally constructed challenges, economic pressures and calls for unpleasant role conformity as fundamental sources of modern mental suffering and distress. He analysed how structural historical conditions placed novel economic demands on new generations of employees and how ethical virtues connected to religion, particularly Protestantism, promoted values that supported laborious behaviour as a key source of salvation (Frommer and Frommer, 1993, 1998). If these structural demands deriving from the economy and culturally produced changes were not met, they were likely to cause numerous problems, including poor mental wellbeing.

In the near history of mental vulnerability, mental health concerns related to work reached new arenas after the Second World War. During an excessive period of rebuilding, a leading German health practitioner, Michael Bauer, developed the concept of *Managerkrankheit* (manager's disease) in the 1950s. He considered it to be a disease of civilization. A lack of sleep, over-taxation of one's capacities, lack of exercise, overwork, the excessive use of stimulants of all sorts and excessive consumer behaviour were the typical symptoms of the disease (Kury, 2017: 63). Many doctors soon came to interpret it as a psychosomatic lifestyle disease, encompassing a wide variety of symptoms, and began to attribute it to the economic and societal situation of the 1950s. According to the Swiss historian Patrik Kury (2017), manager's disease was driven by anxiety and it was manifested in the worryingly high mortality rate among male elites, who were physically and mentally exhausted by the task of rebuilding the country's economy. This historical period connecting the earlier tradition of psychosomatic medicine with current societal changes impacted both the future development of occupational stress research and public understanding of the psychosocial development of disease processes.

The mental vulnerabilities of the first period of modernization had a strong link with social class and the historical challenge of efficiency of work. In the late 19th century, the hectic rhythm of modern life and neurasthenia represented the problems of the higher classes, while 'industrial fatigue' and equivalent problems associated with workers' efficiency worried new groups of organizational managers and work scientists (Rabinbach, 1992). A classic example of paternalism, workplace efficiency and the education of working classes is documented in the letters written by the famous potter Josiah Wedgwood at the end of the 18th century. In the letters, he documented how he continuously wrestled with the organization of work and civilization of workers who had not been used to organized industrial production (McKendrick, 1961). Wedgwood and his various successors intended to combine efficiency and workers' corporeal health, but as Friedrich Engels (2001 [1845]) and some other social critics noted, industrialization provoked a lot of suffering. For instance, the streets of industrial towns of the early 19th century were often occupied by disabled people due to their inhuman work conditions. The mortality and morbidity rates of working-class populations were tragic and became a driving force for later social reforms. In many countries paternalistic work cultures and work communities provided social and environmental contexts for the early development of organizational mental hygiene (Kettunen, 1994), which was a background to the development of occupational psychology and modern protection of employees' psychological health. Today it is well-documented that as the role of industrial production grew, the interest in the psychological wellbeing of the employees gained wider attention among the proponents of the national efficiency movement and work scientists especially since the early 20th century (Blayney, 2019; Mannevuo, 2020).

It can be summarized that the social history of mental vulnerabilities reveals how cultural and economic factors have influenced definitions, etiological descriptions and overall views on stress-related diseases and mental health problems (Liu, 1989; Kury, 2017: 78). Mental vulnerabilities that are today named depression, job burnout, exhaustion, work stress, psychological distress or similar conceptualizations have evident links with the psycho-pathological categories of the earlier historical periods. For instance, the descriptions of acedia and neurasthenia are linked to a lack of appropriate resources, poor capacity to perform valued social behaviours, and psychologically taxing negative moods. The core difference between current mental vulnerabilities and acedia is related to the source of negative mood and low mental energy. Unlike today, the source was typically understood in terms of failure to meet religious expectations, or to live up to duties in the studies on acedia. In turn, the descriptions of neurasthenia already correspond to the nature and etiologic profile of current mental vulnerabilities in many respects. Particularly, symptoms attributed to modern lifestyles, excessive job demands and the contrasts between the adaptive capacity of 'Stone-Age' human bodies and the frantic rhythm of modern society have been seen to underlie various mental vulnerabilities of working-age populations in the past 50 years (Cooper and Dewe, 2008; Väänänen et al, 2012; Schaufeli, 2017).

The ground for the period between the 1960s and 2020s that evidenced a considerable rise in concerns dealing with mental vulnerabilities was built during a lengthy period of modernization of the human sciences, organizations and social behaviour. From the perspective of work and employee health, the seeds of modern thinking on occupational health and safety were sown during the gradual process of industrialization, urbanization and technologization. The differentiated history of vulnerability between the low-educated working population and the modern upper and middle class also shows how mental vulnerability has emerged from different living environments, motives and resources. At the same time, the long history of mental health challenges indicates how similar psychological and emotional challenges have taken place during our documented history. One purpose of this book is to understand why these challenges have become such a large public, social and personal issue, especially in current society and work.

Shifting epidemiologic boundaries

Epidemiological and demographic research on the history of health and mortality can be informative as it has conceptualized the historical changes towards modern diseases. Perhaps the most widely recognized grand model in this domain is called the theory of epidemiological transition (or health transition) (Mackenbach, 1994). This theory was first formulated of epidemiological transition was first formulated in a paper published by epidemiologist Abdel Omran in 1971. It provides a general description and explanation of the spectacular decline first in death rates and then birth rates, which has been observed in all currently industrialized countries. In the epidemiological transition theory, the historical development of mortality over time is characterized by three phases: the 'age of pestilence and famine', the 'age of receding pandemics' and the 'age of degenerative and man-made diseases'. It is the transition from a cause of death pattern dominated by infectious diseases with very high mortality, especially at younger ages, to a pattern dominated by chronic diseases with lower mortality, mostly peaking at older ages, that is seen to be responsible for the tremendous increase in life expectancy (Mackenbach, 1994).

The theory suggests that most of the epidemiological transition has occurred very late in human history along with urbanization and industrialization in the last 300 years. The increase in size of centres of population brought changes in infections, with airborne viruses such as measles and smallpox becoming epidemic where populations were sufficiently large and concentrated. Hence, in the historical accounts of epidemiologists, the transition towards modern society is recognized as an influential factor in the change of human epidemiological environments, and the transition is accordingly explained using nutritional and bacteriological frameworks. It is also repeatedly argued that human beings have evolved for a very different world of hunting and gathering, and adaptation to a modern way of life is still far from complete and causes various physical and mental symptoms (Mercer, 2014: 200).

The history of population health shows how beneficial changes in living environments including work and the extension of public health interventions in the 20th century led to a decline in mortality, while changes in lifestyle and health-related behaviour based on knowledge of risk factors impacted the lay understanding of diseases (Mercer, 2014: 209). As a consequence, a new epidemiological paradigm emerged focusing research on risk factors associated with chronic diseases and older age (Mercer, 2014: 209–210).

Although Omran's theory of epidemiological transition addressed an extremely important global phenomenon, it is also descriptive and poorly developed in terms of human and social sciences. It can be justly argued that the original concept of epidemiological transition oversimplified the changing patterns of disease and causes of death, by viewing them as a replacement of one category by another category of supposedly unconnected diseases (Mercer, 2014: 220). Infectious diseases have their own dynamics and cannot be understood as mental health challenges (or cardiovascular problems). In addition, it has been relatedly shown that not all populations have been able to benefit from technical, economic or social progress, which, theoretically opens a door to a health improvement and to a new step in the health transition (Meslé and Vallin, 2017).

From the perspective of this book, it is striking how theories of epidemiological transition view the change of disease structure from the perspective of physiological and biological conditions, while the transitions in human behavioural patterns and requirements for work capacity remain mainly unrecognized. For instance, the epidemiological transition perspective can say little about why in some contexts emotional and social difficulties are categorized as mental disorders whereas in some other contexts they are left without disease labels. Taking this argument further, among researchers studying cross-national morbidity differences it is well-known that when people are asked to evaluate their own health in materially less developed countries, they draw on their knowledge of what good health means in the context in which they live. In low-income countries the poor will work until they break down partly because taking time off from work is not subsidized in any way except by hard-pressed families who must pick up the slack or suffer the consequences. In this case the term 'cultural' includes how people have learned to identify and respond to less than perfect states of health in conjunction with the amount of institutionalized support they receive for being sick (Encyclopedia of Population, 2019). Hence, the lack of analysis of social dynamics and material reality as well as labour market demands defining and guiding the status and social value of mental vulnerabilities leave the theory of epidemiological transition blind to socially engendered challenges and mental disabilities (Bovet, 2014).

A new epidemiology emphasizes a host of social and behavioural factors that hitherto were not recognized by medical science as a health concern. In the context of 'new health', more and more diseases are not so much 'caught' but 'acquired' (Petersen and Wilkinson, 2008). The association of health with risk is encouraged by the epidemiological understanding that many of the most life-threatening diseases are caused through a combination of multiple 'lifestyle risk factors'. David Armstrong (1995) has interestingly suggested that the language of risk entered the everyday lexicon of medical practice during the period where the imperatives of health moved beyond the treatment of bodily symptoms to work at controlling risk factors in social environments 'implicated within the aetiology of modern diseases of affluence' (Petersen and Wilkinson, 2008). One of the main environments was various conditions of work.

Alan Petersen and Iain Wilkinson (2008: 6) argue that in the late modern societies, the epidemiology of risk led to preventive strategies on a range of fronts from the local level to the individual level. The transition of lay understanding of disease development accompanied the transition towards the epidemiology of risk. Petersen and Wilkinson (2008: 6) even suggest that the self-management of risk has become an imperative of citizenship. 'This entails the close monitoring and regulation of one's thoughts and actions and recognizing oneself as vulnerable.' Based on this, it is possible to make hypotheses related to the changing social behaviour of the population in the area of mental health. For example, increased attention to one's state of oneself may be behind the fact that various expressions of vulnerability have become more common. Be that as it may, this idea shifts the idea of the background of the wounding of the psyche beyond traditional epidemiology to the area of individual and subjective management (Hemmings and Prinz, 2020; Castelpietra et al, 2022; Neufeld, 2022).

The salience of risk conceptualizations can be critically seen as a sign of individualization and the erosion of social ties or as a result of new management strategies that are designed to promote individual's responsibility and activity as 'an organizing ethos of welfare and work' (Petersen and Wilkinson, 2008: 1). It can be suggested that the success of approaches related to adaptation (for example, stress management) and readiness for change (for example, flexibility) in the early decades of the 21st century are examples of this societal transition towards approaches which promote the identification of psychosomatic connections and risk-reducing strategies. These conceptualizations show how the etiological factors and conditions contributing to health have broadened from physiological and biological concerns towards new tactic areas of subjectivity and how the ideal of individual flexibility and risk attentiveness has gained value in the new paradigms of wellbeing.

Particularly since the 1960s, citizens have learned to understand many disease conditions from the perspective of self-made diseases related to poor health behaviours, social conditions or other psychosocial circumstances that could be changed or managed using human-based actions. The problems of mental health and psycho-emotional challenges exemplify these types of 'modifiable conditions' we are accustomed to. It can be argued that in the early 2020s, COVID-19 was a backlash in the long-term subjectivization and individualization of health. When the virus entered our lives with new variants, our collective social compass was confused also because it was not easily modifiable using available procedures and means. This illustrates how we are used to culturally perceiving pathological processes and the nature of disabilities in the labour market and society at large.

Taken together, given the social and changing nature of the psyche and the shift towards less and less material production, the current invasion of mental vulnerabilities cannot be understood using modelling based on bacteriology, virology, physiology or even psychology. But how could the change in social agency be defined and analysed so that the historical nature of psychological ill-health would become more visible?

The birth of autonomous subjectivity

The approaches developed by Norbert Elias (for example, 1991, 1994) and Michel Foucault (for example, 1973, 2005 [1966]) suggest that social researchers should get to grips with the different practices and ways of managing everyday life that have been considered normal and that have changed as societies have developed. If we want to analyse mental vulnerability, we should understand how the recent shift in our socio-emotional activity in a changing society has produced a historically unique way of thinking about and implementing mental health. How might the current mental vulnerability reflect a new late modern ethics of social action and the potential of social characters that perhaps did not yet exist in previous generations?

From this point of view, Canadian social psychologist and sociologist James Côté (2019: 137) has raised an important observation in terms of identity and social expectations among students in Canada and the United States. He emphasizes that only about 20 per cent of young people in the late 2010s had a clear sense of purpose that they could articulate. Côté turns his critical gaze to social character options and psychiatric culture. According to his historical interpretation, previous generations of students understood that going to college involved 'finding yourself', which could be a stressful but also growth-enhancing experience. Currently, he argues, there is a cultural narrative of redemptive therapy that steers students in another direction, into psychological and psychiatric care as a solution. He suggests that many of the observed psychiatric problems in students can be viewed as part of a therapeutic identity narrative that students can adopt when they find themselves overwhelmed by the cross-pressures of higher education. Côté assumes that what in Erik Erikson's (1963) time would have been seen as symptoms of identity confusion have now been medicalized as anxiety and mood disorders, and treatable with medications and therapy. He suggests that in response to the greater availability of psychiatric services, many students may be more likely to come forth with stress and distress as a part of a therapeutic framework that is popular. He also describes that according to the National Survey of Counselling Center Directors from the

US and Canada, in the 1980s, 56 per cent of directors thought that their centre was treating students with more serious psychological problems (Côté, 2019: 144). By 2007, the amount had risen steadily to over 90 per cent of directors and has remained at about that level for the following decade. Côté's interpretation of these results is interestingly structural and does not fully correspond to a simplistic explanation of therapeutic culture. According to him, the therapeutic narratives of students are met with insufficient numbers of positions for young people in the labour market. As many as one half of North American students are experiencing an academic existential vacuum where their own ideals do not meet with the opportunities provided by their education or the reality of the labour market (Côté, 2019: 154). In this situation, both cultural (therapeutic solutions) and socio-economic (lack of adequate work) processes push them towards the broadened framework of mental health. Even though the problem is a societal issue, it is treated as an individual and emotional problem.

Côté analyses the parallel transition between the social character and the decline of the institutional system and economy from the perspective of self-directed identity and the rise of individualism. According to this analysis, Western countries are 'identity societies' in which their citizens need to adapt and cope with various threats to the self. The best profiles of adaptation to identity societies are characterized by high levels of personal agency, self-efficacy and relying on one's inner compass. Intrinsic motivation, purpose for the activities and mental health are words that describe the ideal person (Côté, 2019: 33). This sort of strong intrinsic identity is demanding and based on individualistic ideals and tends to look for psycho-medicalization support.

The concern raised by Côté has relevance also in Europe. People without a sense of continuity, hampered by a poor sense of identity, can exhibit subjective distress and despair. The challenges with direction of the self and the management of one's identity are frequently related to depression and anxiety, which compose the most prevalent outcomes of mental disorders. The loss of the sense of adequate self-control in the social environment pushes individuals' attention and focus on their own bodies and mental problems (Oksanen and Turtiainen, 2005). From this perspective of Western social mentality, the rise of mental vulnerability could be viewed as a historically specific way of forming and affirming identity (Baumeister and Muraven, 1996). From this context, the spread of the mental health crisis can be viewed as a part of a larger trajectory of society which offers dissatisfactory opportunities for the construction of the self and tries to provide ever more individualistic services that could cure these social problems.

The findings by James Côté and some of our findings (for example, Kuokkanen et al, 2013; Anttila and Väänänen, 2015; Väänänen et al, 2019) suggest that various scientific and popular representations reflect a shift in the ideal disposition of a person, from an emotionally controlled and practically skilful person to a socially flexible, adaptable and technologically resourceful character (see also Honneth, 2004; Ehrenberg, 2010) who knows how to use medical and psychological services. The newly emerged social character is not without its problems and needs support. As Sherry Turkle (1997) suggests, participation in new social enclosures and individual-centred demands are associated with a need for continuous validation of the self. 'Who am I? Am I okay? Am I making the right choice here?' From the critical perspective, identity-projects and dilemmas are often framed (for example, Miller and Rose, 2008: 8) as new forms of a governmentality that seeks to produce a notion of a human as an individual with capacities of self-realization and who strives for dignity. For instance, the increasing need for therapeutic support and ethos presents a new form of governing that does not force people to behave in a certain manner, but makes them want to behave in a certain manner for the sake of their own good (for example, Wilkinson, 2009; Brunila, 2012; see also Chapter 4).

A partly different view has been developed by French sociologist Alain Ehrenberg (2010, 2017) who has analysed the development of Western societies. He argues that widespread psychic suffering is distinguished by the idea of not being able to live up the source of expectations, and frequently results in depression, chronic exhaustion and its related syndromes. Behind the symptoms there is fear of loss, difficulties to cope socially and the rise of narcissism. As a background for the vulnerability of the psyche, he identifies three processes in particular: deinstitutionalization, psychologization and privatization of human existence.

Ehrenberg particularly locates the growth of 'mental weariness' in the historical context of the development of human autonomy in the population. He argues that between the 1970s and the 1980s autonomy became the common condition and pervaded social relationships. New populations detached themselves from the restricting local communities and were considered equal citizens. Individual initiative and self-management became highly valued in the workplace where flexible work implies a worker's autonomy. All these changes impacted duties and demands placed on the self. The responsibility of one's agency became a crucial component of existence and highlighted the ability of individuals to be *the agent of their own change*. In this behavioural framework, the subject has to self-control, self-regulate, self-discipline and self-activate, as well as adopt new skills, and all these skills require the perpetual investment of mental energy (Ehrenberg, 2017: 160–161).

Among late modern autonomous subjects, Ehrenberg states that the emphasis is on the problems of self-structuring. Without self-structuring it is difficult to act by oneself in an appropriate manner. This was not a similar concern in the past society of mechanical discipline. At the same time, our existence is ever more frequently formulated in a language of affects and emotions, vacillating between the positive value of mental health and the negative value of psychic suffering. Mental health has become a space where core tensions of our individualism are dealt with and solutions are sought. Consequently, we have seen a change and extension in the social status of psychic suffering. Mental health has occupied a significant role at the scientific (knowledge), institutional (services), organizational (work) and political (decision making) levels. Furthermore, our empirical findings in medical care (Järvensivu et al, 2018; Väänänen et al, 2019; Wilkinson and Väänänen, 2021) indicate how mental health has gradually acquired a value that extends well beyond the area of psychopathology (Ehrenberg, 2017: 162). In line with these ideas, studies show how mental health had quite a marginal role in the management of emotionally difficult situations in the workplace in the earlier stages of modernization (Turtiainen and Väänänen, 2012; Anttila and Väänänen, 2013). This change can be viewed as a transition from a disease-focused narrow psychiatry to the modification of everyday affective states and situations, demanded by current individualist behavioural culture.

According to Ehrenberg, the main difference between traditional psychiatry and modern mental health can be expressed very simply: psychiatry is a local idiom, a specialist in the identification of particular problems. Mental health, because of its very wide spectrum, is a global idiom enabling the formulation of the multiple tensions and conflicts of contemporary life (Ehrenberg, 2017). Being a global idiom, mental health today is intimately embedded in the socialization of the modern individual. According to Ehrenberg, mental health problems arise from the ideals and challenges of an individualist society, such as self-value, the opposition between responsibility and illness, the ability to succeed in work and so on.

Ehrenberg's analysis highlights two major historical changes. The first one is the status of the symptom: a mental problem has become an expression of difficulties related to socialization. Mental health symptoms more and more often reflected the criteria related to performance in work and other arenas of life and difficulties to fulfil the expectations. This was evident in work disability related to mental health that increased considerably more than mental health symptoms in the population. The second change is related to a new cultural dimension of mental vulnerability – unhappiness. Many current manifestations of mental health are related to the feeling of not being able to be good enough, of not being able to mobilize oneself to do things, and the inability to act (Ehrenberg, 2017: 164). If the recent spread of work disabilities related to mental health is considered, Ehrenberg's analysis raises an important conclusion. At the core of the mental vulnerability dilemma lies the dynamic relationship between the cultural change towards individual life management, the transition of health towards challenges produced by autonomous subjectivity and the inadequate socialization of large proportions of populations to the labour market and other recognized social forums providing opportunities for social prestige.

The interpretation that the new form of mental health is related to social behaviour and social behaviour is determined by individual autonomy is essential. In the new idiom, emotional self-control and autonomy are stressed (Ehrenberg, 2010, 2017). In view of this interpretation, it is not surprising that brief and long-term therapies, various techniques of psychological self-maintenance, professional guidelines of mental health and other means supporting autonomous individuals through their various challenges in life and directing the self are at the core of this ethos.

Ehrenberg's analyses provide an interesting view on how psychotherapy has been extended to social problem solving and has often become a form of coaching: social functioning is added to and intertwined with psychopathology. Mental health issues are included in public policies and human resource guidelines, which have larger targets than strictly solving psychiatric problems. They are about how to achieve socialization in a world where the ability to decide and act by oneself pervades social relationships and is the common condition. Mental health is more often the equivalent of good socialization, because being in good mental health is to be able to act by oneself in an appropriate manner in changing social relationships of life (Ehrenberg, 2017: 168–169).

From this perspective, the history of mental ill-health follows a course that runs parallel to the decline in the type of the disciplined individual. The claim is that, since the Second World War, the emancipated individual no longer suffered from the fear of violating social prohibitions, but instead from the exhaustion that sets in as a result of the perceived failure to satisfy requirements. Depression brings to light the difficulties unavoidably faced by an individual who attempts to give himself a structure in a society which attaches supreme importance to personal initiative and self-realization. 'Becoming ourselves made us nervous, being ourselves makes us depressed', Ehrenberg summarizes (see also Wagner, 2017).

Although there have been some differences between affluent economies, the period between the 1970s and 2010s seems to be critical for the invasion of mental health. In Finland and some other rapidly developed countries, the problems with burnout, depression and other similar mental health symptoms started to appear fairly recently (since the late 1970s) and their significance in the everyday lexicon of work and mental healthcare multiplied between the late 1980s and the 2010s. In other words, it seems that the problems of becoming/being ourselves emerged during the era when the late-1900s generations took a central position in the affluent societies.

But how can we empirically study the burden of being ourselves? At least an indirect indicator of the tendency to seek new forms of self-realization and the most satisfactory life contents for oneself can be found in a study of

Finnish working conditions (Sutela et al, 2019), which is the oldest nationally representative European survey assessing changes in working-age populations since 1977. At the end of the 2010s the study showed how nearly two out of three Finnish wage workers saw work as a very important part of their life. According to the study, the 2000s and 2010s saw a significant increase in the role of leisure in employee valuations. However, the home and family life have not lost their role as the most important life arena. To summarize, the importance of all these central areas of life had grown during the early 21st century. The expansion of life areas especially concerns white-collar employees, women and the youngest generations. From the point of view of the structure of the activity, it is reasonable to assume that different spheres of life, competing for resources with each other, clash more and more often. When new areas that consume time and other resources emerge, life can start to feel cramped and choices for 'being ourselves' are needed. Interestingly, organizational research has proposed that pursuing wellbeing or other important individual goals that are, in principle, positive, seems to lead to a reverse result when moving past a certain optimal limit. This has been called the 'too-much-of-a-good-thing-effect' (for example, Busse et al, 2016), but from the perspective provided by Ehrenberg it can be interpreted as a sign of the evolvement of self-content-seeking individuality. The demands of becoming and being oneself have been associated with the increasing importance of different fields of life and as manifestations of the challenge of developing a new autonomous self.

From the perspective of historically changing social character, this can reflect paradoxical processes rising from the dynamic between numerous potential choices, self-focused satisfaction seeking and limited resources available among individuals/employees. In this manner, the spread of problems related to mental health may also signify commitment to the self-related values. A focus on emotionally honest self-structuring of one's life may therefore signify that one is trying to follow a therapeutic behavioural model and intends to manage psychosocial behaviour using mental health support. On the other hand, mental health problems can also reflect poor opportunities to fulfil ego-centred expectations.

Critical organizational research speaks of a 'wellbeing cult' and a 'wellbeing ideology'. They refer to the fact that striving for maximal wellbeing and happiness does not necessarily lead to increased wellbeing, but instead to an increase in the manifestations of unwellness on a societal level (Cederström and Spicer, 2015). Many scholars of cultural history have shown that the status of positive emotions has risen in Western countries, emphasizing happiness and wellbeing, while at the same time increasing the struggle against the counter-pool, depression (Stearns, 1994; Kotchemidova, 2005). According to the critical perspective, the tyranny of positive affect may have stimulated the rise of actions and policies against unproductive and disvalued melancholy and apathy. This may offer one potential explanation as to why the health of the working-age population is better than before in most Western countries, but yet we observe increasing cases of incapacity to work (Ferrie et al, 2014). According to the perspective developed by Ehrenberg, the increase in mental weariness observable over the past 50 years is connected to the rising problems of self-organization, feelings of inadequacy among various populations and the tendency to seek psychological solutions for social problems.

To summarize, it seems highly relevant to reflect on the interconnectivity between the ontology of social character and mental health in different spheres of life. The surge of mental vulnerability in post-industrial society and workplaces is fuelled by strong personal investment in the self-construction of autonomous subjects. The transition in structural conditions for being oneself provides a highly informative approach to understanding the historically unique emergence of mental health concerns. An important contribution is that indicators of mental ill-health are not an outcome of certain risk factors but an essential part of being oneself in current society as being oneself calls for subjective management and mental health frameworks. Simultaneously, the historical-sociological analysis of the change in social agency shows how, for example, psychologization and medicalization were part of the change in both the employee's self and the valued repertoire of actions. It links the historical change in subjectivity to the qualitative shift of the citizenship and workership towards autonomy and the demand for self-management. This provides new keys to understanding the spread of social characters prone to mental vulnerability and links the status of mental health at work as an integral part of the history of modernization.

6

The change in the understanding of occupational health

Occupational health is a key area where the new status and character of mental health in the context of work has been crafted. It has experienced a considerable change due to drastic transition in job requirements, work ability criteria, the occupational health institution and various other areas. It is therefore plausible that materials describing and defining the typical challenges of occupational health in sciences and media can reveal the mechanisms and turning points that contributed to the rise of the phenomenon of mental vulnerability. In addition, the descriptions and views of occupational health professionals who have experienced the emergence of mental health concerns during their work career can contribute to an understanding of the repositioning of mental vulnerability and how it has become part of the work. In this chapter, I shall illustrate how mental vulnerability matured in the occupational health sciences and public discussions about work between the 1960s and 2010s. I also analyse how occupational health professionals, particularly doctors, have been involved in reforming the position of mental health at work and how they view the transition in mental health in the context of changing work.

Crafting stress-fit subjects in scientific forums

Research that explores the social role of scientific knowledge in society has shown how scientific representations and narratives affect our perceptions of health and illness and how we form our understanding of our own and others' mental health (Murray et al, 2003; Morant, 2006). It is therefore important to identify such changes in scientific thinking that may have contributed to the emergence and social development of mental vulnerability at work. From the point of view of the emergence of mental health challenges among employees, I have found it particularly interesting to analyse the widespread and influential research tradition of work stress, in which the mental health of employees has been systematically analysed using scientific methods and theories.

Over the past decades, work stress has been the most studied topic related to mental health at work, providing an explanation of how our Stone Age body has not been prepared to adapt to the demands of modern work. Work stress theory suggests that the mismatch between human psychogenetics and the current state of society fuels stress reactions in the individual and overloads the human mind on a large scale (Newton, 1995; Rose, 1996, 2007; Wainwright and Calnan, 2002; Cooper and Dewe, 2008; Väänänen et al, 2012, 2014). The history of work stress research can reveal how the roots of the concept and narratives on employees' mental vulnerability have progressed in the discourses of stress sciences and how the stimulus-response model, the idea of homeostasis and the body-mind organism burdened by modern work became dominant forms of understanding work-related mental health. It reflects how the views about mental vulnerabilities related to work changed in occupational medicine, work and organizational psychology and psychosocial epidemiology, and what kind of core assumptions about humans the work stress approach has been based on.

To understand the historical advancement of the work stress paradigm we conducted an extensive database search[1] first to define the point in time when the concept of work stress became topical in different disciplines and to examine the frequency it has been referred to in scientific publications (Väänänen et al, 2014). We examined secular trends in scientific publications on work stress, and analysed how a new discursive, institutional, intellectual and subjective space has developed, in which questions related to workers' diminished mental energy became the centre of attention. We found a dramatic rise in the 1980s and the steep increase in the relative share of work stress publications in the scientific databases continued into the 1990s and the early 2000s. Between the 1970s and 2000s, the proportion of work stress publications multiplied both in specialist journals of occupational and public health and applied psychology.

In addition to analyzing quantitative data, we qualitatively analysed a sample of the work stress publications (articles, books, book chapters, unpublished congress presentations, 'state of the art' reviews and book reviews) which were published in the same period. Most of the analysed documents were produced by well-established work stress researchers, and therefore they are likely to represent the legitimized scientific understanding of the work stress phenomenon and the scientific formulation of mental vulnerability in occupational health sciences. We reviewed 132 articles in detail in order to

---

[1] Earlier and lengthier versions of this section have been published in two articles: Väänänen, A., Murray, M. and Kuokkanen, A. (2014). The growth and the stagnation of work stress: Publication trends and scientific representations 1960–2011. *History of Human Sciences*, 27(4), 116–138. Copyright © 2014 by (The Authors). Reprinted by permission of SAGE Publications; Väänänen, A., Anttila, E., Turtiainen, J. and Varje, P. (2012). Formulation of work stress in 1960–2000: Analysis of scientific works from the perspective of historical sociology. *Social Science & Medicine*, 75(5), 784–795. Copyright (2012), reprinted from *Social Science & Medicine*, with permission from Elsevier. I would like to thank the publishers and the other authors for the permission to republish.

recognize how knowledge on work stress gradually took shape, what kinds of assumptions about human nature and work it was based on, and what the aim of this paradigm was.

The first wave of stress studies in the late 1960s and 1970s can be viewed as a part of the broader rational humanization project of industrial work (Väänänen et al, 2012). Often the purpose was to enrich monotonous and machine-dominated work environments and make them psychologically tolerable. For instance, in his seminal work on organizational psychology, *Mental Health of the Industrial Worker*, Kornhauser and Reid (1965) proposed the opportunity to use one's abilities as the most influential positive job attribute related to mental health while haste, intensity and repetitiveness of work operations had adverse impacts. The empirical basis for their analysis was drawn from the Detroit automobile factory context where thousands of industrial employees worked in typical standardized work conditions of that time. William McWhinney and colleagues (1966) brought a wider societal framework to the fore while they positively commented on Kornhauser's and Reid's book in their review: 'One of the important concerns of the humanist throughout the modern era has been with the psychological condition of the worker in the routine, mindless jobs of industry and of the paper-work bureaucracies' (McWhinney et al, 1966).

The development of labour protection and the transition towards reformist values were an important motivational background for many stress researchers in the 1960s and 1970s. In the study of work stress, the humanistic undertone was often combined with the natural science paradigm aimed at objectivity and measurability. Our analyses (Väänänen et al, 2014) revealed that over the course of work stress history, there were some core 'quests' that motivated the surge of work stress research. The first one was the quest to understand emotions at work. During the period under study, work came to be seen by researchers as something that needed to be analysed using psychological and social psychological means, observing the socio-technical environment from the point of view of human mental wellbeing and by applying psychosocial approaches on workers and work communities. The quest was to reduce the psycho-emotional burden and thereby make work more humane and increase productivity. The adverse impact of negative emotions such as stressfulness in the work process became formally recognized by researchers and widely taken as an object of study especially in behavioural and social sciences in the 1970s. Susan Jackson and Christina Maslach (1982), the developers of the burnout concept, described their measures, study findings and the role of emotions in the following way in the early 1980s:

> Recently, a measure was developed to assess human service worker's feelings of personal accomplishment, emotional exhaustion, and

depersonalization (Jackson et al, 1982). Using this measure, we have demonstrated that mental health workers who are emotionally exhausted are perceived by their co-workers as drained by their jobs, and more likely to make negative evaluations of their clients. Emotionally exhausted workers are less satisfied with their jobs, take more frequent work breaks, and have higher rates of absenteeism (Barad, 1979; Jackson et al, 1982). These findings correspond closely to research by others relating feelings of stress and strain to illness, absenteeism, and turnover. (Jackson and Maslach, 1982: 64–65)

Humanist tones started to increase in the scientific understanding of occupational health after the late 1970s. Several authors began to emphasize the need to understand the emergence, development and spread of negative emotions in the workplace and to consider the mental and physical consequences of burdening emotions at work. Instead of concern with exposure to chemical and physical contaminants, the new conceptualizations emphasized the importance of social and emotional factors, both as predictors and as outcomes. At the same time, the role of psychological approaches in occupational health studies grew, focusing on the mental aspects of employees and work communities manifested in stress studies.

Second, at the centre of the corpus of work stress research publications was the quest to clarify the complex relationships between the work environment, the mind and the body, and identify their objective associations (for example, Väänänen et al, 2014). Work stress reviews of the studied era indicated numerous scientifically significant and non-significant associations between different 'factors' (Näring et al, 2006). Work stress publications were often formulated as tests of the impact of the work environment on psychological symptoms, health problems or the risk of some disease. The following extract from the domain of occupational epidemiology illustrates a typical mono-causal approach among work stress scientists:

Results of the conditional multiple logistic regression analysis indicated that stress due to unsuitable jobs was significantly associated with occurrence of major depression after depressive symptoms were controlled for. It is suggested that stress due to unsuitable jobs is a possible risk factor for major depression in industry. (Kawakami et al, 1990: 772)

The extract shows how researchers chose some main explanatory variable and outcome variable and attempted to convince the reader that they had ruled out the potential influence of other stress-inducing factors. This technicalization of phenomenon placed work stress in the concept and mindset of natural science.

The third social need in work stress research was related to the 'quest for balance'. During the period analysed, the importance of the adaptive capacity of the employee's organism when faced with adverse circumstances remained one of the cornerstones of work stress research. The idea of adaptive organism was illustrated in the model of homeostasis by Claude Bernard, which had originally inspired the birth of stress theory (see, for example, Modell et al, 2015). It emphasized the importance of the internal balance of an organism in the face of a changing environment (Cannon, 1932; Kugelmann, 1992). According to stress theory, this 'homeostatic balance' is vital for healthy survival. In the studied documents, work stress was often viewed as consisting of any event in which external or internal demands taxed or exceeded the adaptive resources of the employee, threatening the homeostasis of their body. In the late 1970s, Beehr and Newman (1978: 670), after an extensive state-of-the-art review, defined job stress as 'a condition wherein job-related factors interact with the worker to change (disrupt or enhance) his/her psychological or physiological condition such that the person (mind and/or body) is forced to deviate from normal functioning'.

Although the discourses of work stress subsequently multiplied, and more sophisticated models, attempting to consider contextual circumstances, were developed, the evolutionary paradigm of adaptation of the organism remained central in scientific representations of work stress. A similar observation has also been made regarding the lay representations of work stress (for example, Pierret, 1995; Harkness et al, 2005). However, more political and ideologically critical voices also developed in the work stress literature, and often highlighted the importance of structural and organizational arrangements (organizational changes, reduction in personnel, and so on).

Overall, the steep rise in work stress publications in the 1980s and 1990s reflected growing attempts to gain more knowledge of the ways in which the modern 'psychosocial' work environment might influence the psyche of the new generation of employees (see also Dragus, 1996; Ryder et al, 2002). Simultaneously, other professional approaches stressing the psychological and social dimensions of work grew and mental health-focused organizational consultancies and stress measures were developed to support the psyche (see Koppes, 2007; Warr, 2007). It can be justifiably argued that work stress studies were active promoters of this new psycho-emotional organizational approach characterized by a new kind of human-centred professional knowledge.

Long-term data on the science of work stress offers various interesting interpretative pathways in terms of mental vulnerability in working populations since the 1960s. A 'realistic explanation' for the rise of work stress publications can be found in the structural transition of work. Over the past 50–60 years, typical work in Western societies moved away from physically strenuous and chemically hazardous environments towards new environments characterized by the production or spreading of information and the sale of services. Work stress and mental vulnerabilities related to work could be viewed as rising from the new nature of demands related to the contents and processes of work that are more challenging for the psyche.

A more critical perspective towards work stress points to the growth of emotional management in work (Hochschild, 1979; Anttila et al, 2018; Turtiainen et al, 2022). During the 20th century, there was an increasing trend to pay greater attention to the various emotional aspects of employees, their classification and their more sensitive management (Varje et al, 2013a). The 'work stress turn' in the sciences can be seen as a part of a new economy and production structure that more comprehensively considered the role of the psychological wellbeing of the worker, the successful social interaction, and the positive reactions of the clientele. Interestingly, the steepest rise in scientific work stress concerns in the 1990s also corresponds with the overall intensification of the labour market in Western societies (Green, 2004, 2006). It is not impossible that the higher speed, reduction of 'dead time' and entrepreneurial navigation at work stimulated negative experiences which were often labelled 'work stress', both in lay and scientific representations. It is possible to view the growth of the work stress discourse as arising from attempts to 'manage' the adverse psychosocial consequences of labour intensification in the service/information economy. David Wainwright and Michael Calnan (2002: 197) go even further and claim that the stress discourse has served the purpose of transforming structural labour market conflicts into questions of personal human interaction and individual coping methods and the management of emotions, thus reducing the ability of workers to find politically meaningful responses to the adversities they encounter at work. Indeed, the adaptation of the organism and the quest for inner balance did not have an ideological tone but situated the challenge in the domain of psychobiological functioning.

However, serious attempts were also made to bring the issues related to social inequality and the contextuality of occupational health into the domain of work stress studies (for example, Eakin, 1997). For example, many social epidemiologists who studied inequality placed work-related stress and other 'psychosocial pathways' as a central part of the formation of inequality in mental and physical health (Wilkinson, 2000; Siegrist and Marmot, 2006). Yet the continuous search for various stress-inducing and illness-causing factors remained at the core of work stress research. According to Wainwright and Calnan (2002), epidemiologists specially constructed the 'work stress victim' as a subject within medical discourse, that is, as someone suffering from a disease. In this sense the worker is no longer a political agent struggling for better working conditions, but a vulnerable 'body' to be protected from hazards in the working environment which might cause physical or mental illness.

Because the work stress paradigm formed the most dominant approach in the study of mental health of work, work stress publications can be seen as reflecting the mainstream views on the etiology of work-related mental health in the late 1900s and early 2000s. This leads to a highly important point in terms of mental vulnerability during the heyday of work stress research: by focusing on the immediate environment of work and the employee as an adaptor, many work stress studies naturalized increased psychological intensification. Collective resistance, structural population changes, massive layoffs or the transition towards medical frameworks of behaviour, for instance, did not belong to the fore of work stress thinking characterized mainly by the evolutionary approach and micro-organizational focus (see Young, 1980; Väänänen et al, 2012, 2014). From this point of view, it was also natural from a historical point of view that distress, cynicism or fatigue began to be increasingly understood and treated within the framework of individuals' mental health.

From the perspective of critical psychology, work stress and its siblings can be understood from the social and ideological history of individual-driven constructs. It can be seen to reflect certain ideals and subject requirements that are characteristic for flexible and dynamic markets. Work stress calls for improved adaptivity, inner stability, coping skills and transformative personality traits. These are mostly studied from the perspective of the individual worker. Related to this, there is a long-standing critique of applied psychology which argues that the discipline insufficiently addresses the contextual and cultural nature of the field and its findings. Work stress research has mainly adopted an a-historical and non-cultural orientation which fails to address the way in which both theories and empirical studies reflect the contingent situation of 'a given society at a given moment' (Sullivan, 2020: 94; Newton, 2022).

It is evident that the growth of the work stress approaches closely parallels the overall spreading of medical and psychological frameworks in the domain of work. The rise of work stress was associated with the general medicalization of organizational wellbeing (for example, burnout syndrome, workaholism) and the growing need for psychological frameworks in organizational life (see also Furedi, 2004). So, the general tendencies to medicalize and psychologize social behaviours, emotions and bodily sensations are inevitably present in the scientific making of work stress. However, as Chapter 4 discussed, entirely constructionist perspectives have certain flaws that are related to the overly cultural explanations that give limited attention to changes in the exogenous structural conditions of work (for example, intensification) and/or historical transitions in the general possibilities and limits of social behaviours (for example, 'democratization' and 'civilization' of social relations). It seems evident that both the change in the labour market and the change in the structural perspective of the subject have pushed phenomena such as work stress to the fore.

The development of work stress research can be placed in the change of the historical landscape of the psyche in the maturing welfare democracies, where an individual's responsibility over their own health was increasingly promoted (for example, health) (Crawford, 1994; Murray et al, 2003). Scientific knowledge about work stress started to provide more tools for managing individuals' psychological issues and it started to have a political function. In the same way as the new middle-class health consciousness emphasizing mental fitness may have looked for autonomy, power and moral integrity through the achievement and maintenance of a hard body (exercise, asceticism) (Ehrenreich, 1989; Crawford, 1994; Shilling, 2002), so may have the management of occupational stress in the domain of a working mind.

The work stress representations from the late 1960s until the 2010s can be interpreted to reflect a new form of 'occupational health consciousness', emphasizing the role of an autonomous character, who perseveres through stressors and other psychological challenges using various individual and microsocial coping strategies. Especially since the 1980s the proactive coper and successful manager of one's emotional life became an ideal organizational citizen. Thousands of scientific work stress documents promoted this perspective by identifying practical ways of coping with harmful stress. At the same time, critical observations were made arguing that opportunities for self-management and coping were not equally distributed. For instance, Mildred Blaxter (1976) argued that 'there are many groups in the population whose position in the social structure makes it difficult for them to subscribe to that belief in the rational mastery of the world which typifies the professional approach'.

Our analyses on work stress trends show that both the absolute and relative growth in research activities focusing on work stress increased towards the end of the 20th century and continued to grow in the early 2000s. More recent data shows that the peak of work stress publications has been reached in various sciences. A heterogeneous set of conceptualizations now increasingly characterizes the current state of art in the field, including concepts such as 'work–family balance', 'recovery from work', 'boredom', 'work engagement', 'psychosocial risks', 'resilience', and so on. There seems to be an increased tendency for researchers to examine more specific issues that fall under or have stemmed from the work stress rubric. This pluralization of the mental vulnerability field probably forms a part of the development in which scientific frameworks and risk observations are increasingly characterizing our daily social lives and collective understanding. In this respect, the recent invasion of various approaches to wellbeing in occupational health and organizational studies does not present anything new.

Instead, the transformation of the risks of negatives into risks of positives occurs in a similar microcosm to work stress studies.

Generally, the scientific documents of work stress formed an important part of the production of socio-cultural representations of occupational health among the new generations of employees after the late 1970s. These representations were mostly related to the immediate work content (for example, job strain, role ambiguity) or individual's capacities (for example, social support, self-efficacy) to cope with this adverse 'psychosocial environment'. In this manner, studies of work stress gradually transformed the epidemiological model based on chemical, physiological and biological exposures to the world of social and psychological features characterized by interaction, shared meanings and subjective experiences. These analyses understood social and psychological environments as containing potential exposures ('risks') that can be detected using validated instruments and used to identify the vulnerable subjects and groups in the working-age population.

In conclusion, the shift in science towards concern about work stress can be interpreted as one part of a new way of understanding work, production and employees' roles in them. According to our analyses, the work stress literature expanded when the nature of work processes, the basic outcome of work, and the whole culture shifted towards non-material aspects, an information focus and need to organize social relations. The growth of work stress research was stimulated by the intensification and the increasing importance of the emotional sphere of the labour market. It also seems likely that the 'work stress turn' was characterized by a shift towards new subjective experiences among the growing segment of white-collar employees, surrounded by the 'psychosocial' environment, and characterized by self-management. The larger cultural and economic shift required novel approaches able to conceptualize and provide information regarding late modern work and the vulnerability of workers. As one of the key life-structuring representations of late modern work, 'work stress' absorbed various unpleasant characteristics of modern work.

In this way, historical studies on work stress expand the discussion on the rise of mental vulnerabilities by showing how work stress studies' scientific assumptions and social role are connected to changing societal and organizational needs. While the representations draw upon everyday experiences of distress in the workplace, they also scientize them, and aim to make them controllable within a rather specific engineering framework. Within this framework, the impact of adverse working conditions (such as production overrun) or the consequences of structural macro-level changes (such as global recession) is easily perceived from the perspective of the individual's mental health/abilities. From this perspective, it is not surprising that occupational mental health research has been criticized for being medicalized and psychologized as well for having an uncritical attitude towards discourses that make the individual responsible of their self-management. Simultaneously, the history of work stress research shows how the dominant human character in occupational health research was positioned within the framework of individual-centred mental health and biology-driven human image over several decades.

Work-related mental health in the media discussion

Media discussions are an obvious part of the culture that produces and structures vulnerability. It is therefore important to find out how the change towards the new work, labour market and perhaps the new employee character understood in psychosocial terms was reflected in the changes of the public debate about work and occupational health. As historical documents, media documents representing a long period of time provide valuable materials on typical views and perceptions of work, its challenges and occupational health. They also reveal how descriptions and views on the demands of work and discussions on mental health altered as society and work changed.

This chapter describes how the media portrayed work and work-related psychological burdening in the society living through a strong phase of change. How did the awareness of mental vulnerability possibly arise in the media? How did the discussion in the media change the depictions of work and the employees' required abilities? What kind of behaviour was seen as desired and valuable in terms of occupational health and psychological work ability in different times?

With historian Pekka Varje[2] (Varje and Väänänen, 2016), I investigated the long-term changes in occupational health discourses and descriptions of common problems faced by employees at work. Using archival data, we studied how psychosocial risks and mental strains of work were discussed in the media in Finland from the 1960s to the late 2000s. We also analysed the occupational health discussions from the perspective of social class transition because in Finland the phenomenon was associated with a strong transition from manual and heavy work to offices and services, which meant a change in the culture and values of social classes in addition to work tasks. The source material of the article was drawn from two Finnish publications. *Helsingin Sanomat* (HS) is the largest daily published newspaper in Finland, while

---

[2] An earlier and lengthier version of this section has been published in Varje, P. and Väänänen, A. (2016). Health risks, social relations and class: An analysis of occupational health discourse in Finnish newspaper and women's magazine articles 1961–2008. *Sociology of Health & Illness*, 38(3), 493–510. I would like to thank the publishers and Dr Pekka Varje for the permission to republish.

Me Naiset (MN) by the same publisher is the largest weekly published women's magazine. The two publications were selected because they are among the most widespread mediums through which occupational health discussions are introduced to non-specialized audiences. The newspaper and magazine articles used as the source base offer a longitudinal view of the occupational health discussions as they appeared to lay audiences. They reflect concerns and topics about occupational health and are likely to influence the audience and their perceptions of psychosocial risks and mental vulnerabilities in the workplace (Fusco, 2006; Brownlie, 2011).

First, we found that the attention to psychosocial risks during the 1960s and 1970s was relatively adventitious. However, the organization of work, especially of repetitive work in industrial plants, caused some worry about exhaustion and other health problems especially in the 1970s. Occasional attention was also paid to the social relations, efficiency requirements and mental strain:

> In a work environment, competition often causes mental health problems. A few factories experimented switching from a piecework rate to equal pay and a fixed salary. Contrary to the beliefs of the management, the production levels increased rather than decreased, because the stress and tension caused by the competition were replaced by enjoyment of work. (MN, 5 January 1972)

In the 1980s, there was a major turnaround in the discussions on psychosocial health risks at the workplace. In HS, which had earlier largely neglected psychosocial risks, there was a major quantitative change: during the three decades from the 1980s to the 2000s, psychosocial risks were addressed in 28 of 53 articles dealing with occupational health. In MN, the corresponding numbers were 15 out of 23. There was also a major qualitative change. The psychologically burdening aspects of the workplace became problematized, and new measures were called for. This quote from the mid-1980s reveals how the new phenomenon of burnout was approached:

> If several people at a workplace start suffering from burnout, the problem, according to the experts, is in the whole organization. This for its part requires changes, the kinds that cause resistance. … Of course, this does not mean that an individual worker should not check their own attitude, ways of thinking and values from time to time. (MN, 17 September 1985)

According to our analysis, there was a strong linkage of the reported representations of mental vulnerability with the transition of occupational structure and the new emerging economy. As the balance of occupational structure shifted from industrial to clerical and white-collar jobs, a new discourse developed in the public media. A new sensitive tone towards mental health and wellbeing meant that social conflicts, previously seen as natural parts of a hierarchical order of work, were detached from social structures. They came to be presented as potential workplace- and individual-related threats to wellbeing that disrupt the natural order of occupational health and cause psychological suffering to individuals. Previously mostly unofficial micro-social environments and subjective experiences were transformed as crucial elements of occupational health.

The analysis of social/occupational class provides a highly important perspective for understanding this transition. It seems that the new occupational health discourse interested in the subjective states of employees and psychosocial environments such as a good social atmosphere or job control was based mostly on an idealized image of the middle-class workplace presented in the media as the universal model for the healthy and wellbeing-focused workplace. Unlike in the 1960s and 1970s, post-1970s occupational health articles disregarded questions of class but also started to push working-class means of coping with threats to their freedom and dignity, such as strikes, towards the margins of discussion. The key contradiction in the critical articles was that society's harmony was frequently damaged by the culture of competition and inequality creating human and social suffering. In the media texts of the 1980s and 1990s the worry about mental health and social problems often stemmed from the mismatch between the idealized middle-class expectations and the market liberalism focused on producing more profits and increasing efficiency. Especially during and after a deep recession in the 1990s, the newspaper and magazine articles painted a grim picture of the mental health situation in the Finnish labour market, plagued by stress, burnout and a variety of psychiatric problems:

> Burnout has turned out to be more common in Finland than expected … over half of the working population experience some level of burnout, and roughly 165,000 cases of burnout are serious. Every fifth worker is constantly very tired, and seven per cent suffer from impaired occupational self-esteem and have become cynical. Work no longer brings pleasure and has lost its meaningfulness. (HS, 30 October 1997)

At the same time as the economy and labour markets were penetrated by a global market economy ideology, occupational health debates increasingly adopted a strong thought model that regarded the harmony of interests as a desired state, where it was appropriate to reach welfare equations that benefit both employees and employers. Simultaneously, the public discourse of work-related health extended far beyond any physical or biological definitions of health. Besides the image of the healthy worker, the studied articles began to redefine the image of the ideal worker. They glorified a co-operative, organization-friendly behavioural model and active organizational citizenship. Emotional regimes were defined in which every participant in the workplace community is responsible for the managerial tasks of strengthening the positive atmosphere at the workplace, building ties between superiors and subordinates, and actively contributing to the endeavours of the organization. Psychological challenges at work were associated with work-related pathologies that could be prevented by developing psychosocial dimensions of the workplace and fine-tuning one's own behaviour to match workplace ideals. This also marks an interlacing between occupational health discussions and management theories. The idea was not new, as group affiliation, commitment, emotional sensitiveness, teamwork and closer relations between workers and superiors are themes that many organizational theorists have been proposing since the 1930s in order to reduce unwanted behaviour and promote productivity (Barley and Kunda, 1992; Guillén, 1994; Seeck, 2008). 'Investment in good leadership yields multiple returns. At best it improves efficiency and the fluidity of labour, the clarity of responsibilities, know-how and innovativeness, commitment and motivation, good atmosphere, health, and work ability' (HS, 25 September 2007).

Our datasets show how, since the 1980s, the discourses and narratives typical in the media documents worked to assimilate personal emotions with organizational power and generate new social characters who consider the emotional involvement and commitment a reward (Barley and Kunda, 1992). This tendency towards emotional and human-centred perspectives has also been observed in other analyses concerning the long-term development of journalism (for example, Schmidt, 2021). So, it seems that the turn towards competitive white-collar organizations and new cultures of wellbeing at work was manifested in the development of discourses on stress and exhaustion and a new psychosocial organizational language. These kinds of perspectives and concepts were likely to be attractive in the eyes of the media and the readers because they were able to reduce the arbitrariness of psychic and social suffering but gained a more manageable form through scientific explanations. It has been also argued that these perspectives borrowed from science were applied as ideological tools for redefining questions of social risks and individual responsibility (Pollock, 1988).

However, from the perspective of social subjects, one of the problems with these arguments is that they leave us uncertain about whether the subjectivity of the worker is transformed through the discourse or whether workers are able to find means of resisting the discursive power (Bolton, 2005: 42). This problem can be further elaborated by taking note of the fact that the audience of the media discourse is not uniform and consists of people in different social positions who have different experiences. Those who belong to the rising middle classes may find the occupational health discussions to be a confirmation of what they already believe is right and what their personal experience suggests. Those in less advantaged positions who experience work as unfair may find the discussions false, repulsive or simply uninteresting. As Bourdieu (1984: 199) argues, what is distinguished and respectable to middle-class representatives may be pretentious and false to working-class members, and what is straightforward and real to the working classes may be vulgar or shameful to the middle classes. The difference is that the dominant classes are more likely to establish their manners, tastes and codes as the legitimate standard about proper emotional behaviour models against which all other models are compared.

Most media documents studied were presented as universal descriptions about work. The image of the psychosocially healthy workplace in the media did not specify the type of workplace, the kind of work that was done there, or the class or gender that was being addressed. Since the 1980s, the discussions were often characterized by the ideals of classlessness and win-win situations that have gained currency. The market-driven focus on the individualistic strive for social rewards and organizational wellbeing (McDonald and O'Callaghan, 2008) delegitimized the kind of acceptance of conflict and hierarchy that even a women's magazine could still portray in the 1960s and 1970s. From this perspective, the need for harmonious workplace solutions in a competitive environment are intimately related to the transition of occupational health towards psychological concerns and mental health problems (see also Harvey, 2005; Burawoy, 2012).

The publications showed that the idea of the employer as a threat to workers' freedom and a factor calling for a strong counterculture among workers was not at all as common as it used to be. The new paradigm proposed that with the appropriate configuration of democratic leadership and employee engagement, productivity would increase, and worker efforts would be rewarded – there would be no need for feelings of being deceived or otherwise put down. To guarantee the smooth operations of the healthy organization, free flow of information should be enabled, hierarchical conflicts should be worked out, and a debate about employees' experiences should be started.

The rise of the new work culture also meant a fundamental change in the descriptions of the structure of health and wellbeing. In the new media discussion, a more active employee ideal emerged. According to these views, a worker who builds trust within the organization and successfully nurtures innovation and information streams is highly valued and respected. The worker who does not live up to the standards is a potential organizational risk and a cause of unproductivity; and without productivity there will be no rewards that guarantee mental wellbeing and other subjective rewards. This approach departed from working-class behavioural modes and defines them as unwanted. In this manner, the transition of occupational health discussions reveals how the spreading of new middle-class norms was connected to new cultural ideals on active individuals and dynamic workplaces. In the media, this also meant that there was more discussion about the psychology of work communities and the personal wellbeing management of individuals.

The ideals of the wellness-oriented middle-class character with the intention to evolve psychological capacities and resources have been related to the rise of psychological humanism and humanistic psychology in Western societies (for example, Maslow, 1968). In our recent archival study in which we used another major women's magazine, *Eeva*, as a data source we analysed the development of ideas representing humanistic psychology (Nordberg, 2022). The historical data indicated that topics related to finding oneself, self-realization and self-development increased from the 1970s and became highly popular by the end of 20th century. It was clear that the articles in the magazine began to highlight a character who acted proactively using psychological self-observation and listening to one's own self. This new character was self-developing and future-oriented. The core of the character was based on the dynamism and flexibility of the psyche. The emphasis on mental health fitness was thus part of a broader shift in the cultural character ideal.

New humanistic classless norms gained wider readership and popularity, especially among the audience of women's magazines between the 1970s and early 2000s. It seems likely that the spreading of these new ideas in society was accompanied by the increase in mental health concerns because overcoming psychological hardships and emotional crises was an intimate part of the self-developmental narrative. In the articles, mental health was either indirectly or directly present. In media texts, the cure was often found in the evolvement of emotional maturity and psychological growth. But the change was not only related to how employees were seen. The new production structure, work culture and intensifying competition brought out a new social character. This character was required to have psychological qualities and an entrepreneurial business-orientated attitude. Mental endurance and mental wellbeing were organic parts of the development of this social character.

The historical transition of the social character and the rise of work-related wellbeing in media texts offer important clues of the interrelationships between the change in social values, individualization of work and spreading of novel vulnerabilities in a culture in transition. Media texts also underly the intimate connection between the rise of middle-class ideals, psychosocial work discourses and self-developmental ideals. The fundamental power-distances and inequalities characterizing societies based on social hierarchies, including the Finland of the 1950s and 1960s, underwent a process of corrosion from the 1970s onwards. The birth of a new socio-cultural space and discourse with apolitical character in the media reflected a significant change in the way employees, their workplaces and occupational health were portrayed and positioned in the publicity. It is evident that the transition towards psychological challenges and self-caring individualism also resulted in creating a broader ground for the rise of mental vulnerabilities.

The entry of the reflexive character in occupational healthcare

The earlier research materials in this chapter, science and media texts, reflect long-term changes at the public level. However, the analyses of public views, explanations and desired objectives often lead to rather general analyses and assumptions regarding social mechanisms dealing with medicalization, psychologization, individualization and other similar processes. For instance, public texts are not able to provide us with a view on how employees as patients and their interactions with health professionals changed or how health professionals have experienced the changes that the media brought up.

There is a need for information from the grassroots level of crafting mental vulnerabilities in the domain of work and disability that would cover a sufficiently long period of time. Next, I will present results from an interview study on the insights of doctors and other health professionals who had experienced a period of drastic societal transition in Finland through their work.[3] Their descriptions and interpretations are important in order to understand the changing role of mental health challenges in the context of work and how they have been tackled in the healthcare practices concerning employees and their disability.

With my colleagues I gathered data using in-depth interviews (Väänänen et al, 2019; Varje et al, 2021; Wilkinson and Väänänen, 2021). In countries with exclusive occupational healthcare for the employed – such as Finland (Martimo and Mäkitalo, 2014) – occupational health physicians and other occupational health professionals play a vital institutional role in caring and managing employees' mental health problems, because the vast majority of the working population uses occupational healthcare when they encounter challenges of health and work ability. Occupational health doctors especially draw lines between work ability and disability and evaluate the underlying

---

[3] Earlier and lengthier analyses on this topic have been published in two articles: Väänänen, A., Turtiainen, P., Kuokkanen, A. and Petersen, A. (2019). From silence to diagnosis: The entry of the mentally problematic employee into medical practice. *Social Theory & Health*, 17(4), 407–426; and Wilkinson, I. and Väänänen, A. (2021). The informalization of doctor–patient relations in a Finnish setting: new social figurations and emergent possibilities. *Sociology of Health & Illness*, 43(9), 1965–1980. I would like to thank the publishers and the other authors for the permission to republish.

reasons for employees' sicknesses (OECD, 2010). In this way, occupational health doctors and other professionals of occupational healthcare present a continuation of the practice of industrial medicine with a good view of the occupational environment and the challenges of work of their patients compared to other health professionals.

Our research materials indicated a strong and large-scale cultural change that entered the clinic along with the patients' changing problems and ways of working. For example, there was an increasing willingness to express difficult feelings to a doctor and to interpret one's own problems using diagnostic language. The change meant changing the role of the doctor to that of a professional interlocutor, who interprets the client-patient's situation through interaction and supports him or her in emotional and social challenges. According to our results, it appears that as these doctors and other health professionals sought to better accommodate and manage the problems that patients submitted to them for diagnoses, they were being moved towards a greater recognition of the determining influence of wider social conditions over occupational health problems and upon their role and identity as health professionals. Thus, the historical transition of the social character not only involved patients but also health professionals and their behaviour. The practice of medicine under conditions of informalization, which meant more informal and more interactive patient–doctor relationships, emphasized the need for doctors to understand the new challenges of mental health from the perspective of societal change. The development entailed a heightening consciousness of the social forces shaping both the symptoms of disease and diagnostic interpretations concerning psychological challenges.

While occupational health professionals' interpretations of the social sources of patients' psychological problems may be valued as a way of making sociological and cultural sense of the increasing incidence of a society's mental health problems, the increasing intentions to solve the problems produced by the social world in a medical framework also invite me to speculate over the extent to which mental vulnerabilities are the result of a reconfiguration of the relationships between doctors and their emotionally informed patients. Insofar as these are made more subject to processes of informalization in medical encounters and health services, then we might also expect the expression and documentation of experiences of social distress to become more culturally elaborated and widespread.

The spreading of issues that are considered mental health challenges also signified the emergence of new discursive and institutional arenas in which solutions were mutually sought in an atmosphere of openness. It was increasingly common to be accompanied by a doctor, psychologist or short-term therapist. This observation corresponds with the democratization process in other spheres of life in formal social settings, such as in classrooms (Anttila and Väänänen, 2015). This was related to the rise of the educational level in the population as well as the renewal of cultural codes of behaviour. When people needed to reflect their feelings and patterns of behaviour and mental wellbeing became a lifegoal, doctors were required to have more expertise of the psyche as well. Simultaneously, the doctor's position as an authority figure diminished and their expertise became challenged in various ways (Löyttyniemi, 2001).

It seems that especially since the 1990s the role of the patient became more active because of the widespread societal expectation that people should take an active part in managing and surveying their own health (Rose, 2007; Wouters, 2007). In this new 'social figuration', difficulties in working and personal life were understood as something that needed medical or psychological care and consultation (cf Ehrenberg, 1991). It seems that the proliferation of the internet strengthened this process and paved the way for increased awareness of psychological distress.

'There is a terrible load of social problems that people expect doctors to solve that do not, in a sense, concern them. It's become more and more difficult. Then when authority is dismantled, there are many different opinions: Google, the press, the radio. … Yes, nowadays patients have many sources of this kind, people can ask for advice here, there and everywhere, and then choose the answer that suits them best.' (Male doctor, born in 1951, started practising in the 1970s)

In our materials, many interviewees saw this expressive individuality as a latent factor that had induced the recognition of emotional worries and even the emergence of experiences of vulnerability. Doctors commented that people expressed themselves using a "language of injury" and used dramatic expressions such as "I panicked when he/she asked that" (female doctor, born in 1957). The doctors' remarks were similar to the argument that the discourse on psychological hurt and therapeutic remedy has become a powerful cultural paradigm, within which people narrate and construe their lives (McLaughlin, 2011). Overall, our results suggest a close interrelationship between decreasing social hierarchies between doctors and their patients, changing behavioural codes related to psychological suffering, and the altering of strategies for coping with mental distresses.

'The biggest change is that when I started as a physician in the 60s and 70s the medical doctor was an important figure. The patient didn't come to the consultancy with a completed diagnosis, but he/she came to seek advice and with certain symptoms. Then it was easy to give instructions and people believed them and acted accordingly. But now people come in with a Google diagnosis … [Earlier] it was more about the trust and using the methods you had in hand. … Perhaps it was easier for both parties involved, I think.' (Male doctor, born in 1941, started practising in the 1960s)

The spreading of the mental health domain signified a shift from a biomedical to a psychosocial perspective, characterized by a pronounced interactive component. This process has led to a new situation: although the number of clinically diagnosable severe mental illnesses stayed on pretty much the same level over the period 1980–2010, the amount of people suffering from various mental health problems often labelled as 'mood disorder', 'acute stress reaction', 'panic disorder' and 'moderate depression' radically increased. As psycho-emotional difficulties were hard or impossible to approach using traditional methods of medical examination, examination has increasingly relied on discussion, listening and observing the patient's habitus.

The interviews revealed the growth of a more equal distribution of psycho-medical knowledge in the doctor–patient relationship. The shift towards a shared treatment decision-making model (Charles et al, 1999) in the domain of mental health problems also made the role of the medical professional more ambivalent. The medicalization of lay views on mental health problems challenged professionals' work in healthcare. But as the recognition of the problems grew, the awareness of the limitations of medical knowledge and expertise in the face of the phenomenon of psychological vulnerability grew as well. This, in turn, also led to pressures to reduce and limit medicalization (see also Halfmann, 2012). In our studies, the weakening of the mental ill-health stigma was closely linked to the shifts in the social codes of behaviour and the decline of the narrow 'insanity' definition of mental ill-health in the public understanding.

Our research material shows how the new emotional regulation based on informal expressiveness and open reflection of one's feelings was promoted as a 'feeling rule' among the new generation of employees (see Wouters, 2007). The increased recognition of mental disorders among occupational health professionals was intertwined with the codes of emotional management of individuals and the cultural norm of the self-caring citizen (Bröer and Besseling, 2017). New mental problems requiring treatment entered the medical arena and were often unspecific and unidentifiable through clinical examination.

Our interviews indicated that many doctors were consciously adapting their clinical practice and their diagnostic vocabulary in a bid to better manage a new range of mental health problems. The medical profession was actively and consciously involved in creating a conceptual language to render these more subject to terms of medical control and treatment. Moreover, some of our respondents welcomed the new opportunities they had to create a new range of cultural codes and social spaces for their patients to vent their psychological strains on the understanding that this represented a new advance in rendering them formally recognizable as illnesses. For example, one of the doctors describes the transition in the following way:

'We started to have problems in the domain of mental health. We decided to conduct a Bergen Burnout Inventory for all employees. This was in the mid-2000s. Clear cases of burnout were indicated. Some were previously unknown. I interviewed them all. Typical symptoms were a lowered sense of professional efficacy and cynicism. Earlier they would not have dared to come to a doctor. It was quite exciting that after we started to perform the burnout inventory they started to come to the appointments – it somehow turned on the tap.' (Male doctor, born in 1951, started practising in the 1970s)

The occupational health arena experienced a great wave of psycho-emotional problems that were not even recognized as such in earlier decades. As a consequence, more psychological expertise was called for, especially from the 1990s onwards.

'In the corporation we have a workplace programme with an associated "wellness at work" website. And we have also written a job satisfaction guide in which there are sections on recovery, stress and the work community issues. … Then there is the "let's talk about work" model that is our early support preventative model, according to which the foremen are trained and there is support for them with respect to supporting their subordinates, and support for the foremen's own coping is also included.' (Female doctor, born in 1954, started practising in the 1970s)

In the interviews, the perceived transition was that of an ideal employee/patient from a down-to-earth person to a psychologically reflective character who doctors welcomed with mixed feelings. It seems plausible that the proliferation of the middle classes opened a space for a discursive revolution from the late 1970s (Väänänen et al, 2012; Varje and Väänänen, 2016). This was clearly manifested in the growth of debates related to subjectivity and its (psychological) problems. The change was also accompanied by a scientific transition. It is not a coincidence that the steep rise of work stress discourse in several Western countries took place in the media (Wainwright and Calnan, 2011) and in scientific scholarship (Väänänen et al, 2014) during the same period.

Our interview material is to some extent in accordance with the argument concerning consumerism among patients, suggested by findings in the United States (Moloney, 2017). In the new framework, the care of employees' wellbeing and mental health is seen as part of a wider societal change related to customer-orientedness and the development of customer-oriented services. For instance, Google-diagnoses and active seeking of the 'right opinion' was mentioned (healthcare as a marketplace), but on the other hand, patients' active suggestions concerning certain psychotropic medical treatment were seldom noted. Echoing some previous research, several doctors described transitions in patient comportment, self-expression and related behaviours as being fuelled, at least partly, by media attention to mental health (Brown et al, 2015). It is evident that the opening of the public space to the psyche and the processing of emotions has paved the way for discussing mental health topics in a medical context and the treatment of mental health in occupational healthcare has become more accepted. Mentally self-observant and emotionally worried employees entered the medical arena as the transition took place in the health discourse and cultural norms of emotionality (Schmidt, 2021) as well as the behavioural repertoire of work.

Our research illustrates a transition from the culture of social hierarchies and silence of psychological problems towards the 'collective emancipation of emotions' that accompanies a fast relaxation of 'formalized' manners and codes of self-restraint (Wouters, 2007: 202, see also Wouters, 1986, 2011). What was ignored or not even seen as a problem got a new kind of interpretative context when the late modern framework of emotional activity developed and fostered the development of a new mental health. For individuals, this was often desirable, as they had to wrestle with the new demands of emotional management and self-organization. Both doctors and their patients acted in a late modern context where rules of etiquette are rendered more flexible, codes of behaviour made more varied and the individual psyche becomes more subject to conflicts and uncertainty. The stressed and depressed subjects worried about their emotional state but with new abilities moved towards medical and psychological discourses and encounters to seek solutions. According to this interpretation, as power distances were lowered and codes of emotional conduct became more flexible, the mental health domain transferred into a legitimate arena in which employees as customers and individuals increasingly sought solutions for their difficulties.

Interestingly, related observations about the change in the work of occupational health professionals can be seen in other analyses of the same era. The informalization of occupational life and lowered hierarchies have been recorded in our other studies. With the erosion of the traditional social order of the workplace, social interaction skills, psychological capabilities and versatile stress tolerance have come to the fore, as we have tried to reach themes that have emerged since the 1950s (Kuokkanen et al, 2013, 2020; Varje et al, 2013a; Varje and Väänänen, 2016; Anttila et al, 2018; Väänänen et al, 2019; Turtiainen et al, 2022). In many areas of the labour market, the loosening of social hierarchies (for example, teachers versus pupils, doctors versus patients, supervisors versus subordinates or social workers versus welfare recipients) has created a need to address the problems of subjectivity in a professional way (through stress management, therapy and so on) and to solve problem situations in a civilized manner (through negotiation, programmes, counselling and so on).

Thus, the informalization encouraged professionals to adopt a more democratic and considerate attitude towards their clients but it also changed the role of the employees and encouraged increased expressions of subjective views and active seeking of advice and support. This dialogical development put great demands on emotion management skills of various professionals, thereby impelling them to adopt an emotionally sensitive approach in their work. In summary, the modernization and civilization of work communities and of society in general have paved the way for greater mental reflection, psychological support and new practices regarding vulnerability in late modern work. Drawing from the process of informalization and its consequences, the surge of mental vulnerability can be interpreted as a part of a general social change in the post-Second World War era. This does not mean that work-related demands are irrelevant to the surge of mental vulnerabilities, but these results emphasize the importance of other enabling social mechanisms underlying the historical emergence of mental vulnerabilities.

In the analyses stressing the processes of psychologization and medicalization, these historical transitions affecting the fundamental structure of social behaviour, related to changes in power relations, organizational codes or work tasks, have often remained poorly recognized. In turn, in psychological studies on work-related health, this temporal change that shaped the entire research object has often been neglected and the roots that generate the activity understood as mental health do not come to the fore. Based on our analyses, I argue that if we want to understand the spectacular rise of mental vulnerabilities, I see it as essential to understand the change in the 'composition' of the social character and emotional behaviour over a long period of time in different spheres of life.

This conclusion suggests that there is a need to analyse various historical shifts impacting the management of emotions and psychological states as well as the order of mental health in various sceneries of institutional and social life. This signifies that there is a need to look at different, seemingly unrelated processes affecting the centrality of mental health – or more precisely – problems that are located and labelled as mental health challenges in todays' organizational and healthcare practices. They are not found by looking at the epidemiological explanations, stress management guidelines, women's magazines or occupational health debates but these kinds of materials can provide important information on the ingredients contributing to the rise of mental vulnerabilities in our culture.

7

The historical pathways of mental vulnerability in different occupations

Social research focusing on medicalization, psychologization, individualization and intensification has been criticized for presenting the workers as almost invisible objects of the process with little agency of their own (for example, Bolton, 2005). Most analyses do not include questions of how subjectivity in relation to vulnerability has changed, what interests the workers may be pursuing in the formation of their identities, and whether there is in fact a body of workers who can be subjected to such universalizing knowledge at all. 'The worker remains a transhistorical and cultural object who is ever-present but never defined', as social theorist Chris Shilling puts it (see Shilling, 2003: 69–72). If we take this idea to the empirical level, we should investigate different groups of employees in their organizational circumstances and identify essential transitions and characteristics in their work. To understand the current role of mental health in work, we need information about workers in different occupations.

In this chapter, I analyse how mental vulnerabilities have emerged in distinctive areas of work and how they reflect historically specific dialogical structures and behavioural options in which social behaviours and emotions are formed, shared and relived. Through the archival study of insurance sector employees, teachers' work and social work, I intend to clarify how the vulnerability of the mind became a problem, which was seen to erode work ability, and how the change in society was associated with these partly separate historical paths.

The shifting role of mental health problems in the insurance sector

The private business sector forms one of the core areas of economy both in terms of the number of employees and its economic significance. The insurance sector is one of the typical business sectors which has developed through technological transitions and changes in labour markets over the past decades (OECD, 2017). In countries with rapid societal modernization, employee relations within this industry and the work itself have experienced considerable changes along with urbanization and intensification. Insurance employees have typically faced organizational turmoil, layoffs and various changes because companies have had a need to adjust to new economic environments and reduce organizational inefficiencies in more competitive business ecosystems (Knights and Willmott, 1995). For instance, in Finland, the period from the 1960s to the 2010s saw a drastic transition in the organization of work, leadership and distribution of work roles. At the same time, the insurance sector represents an occupational environment that has consistently been highly service-oriented and subject to the interactional characteristics and challenges of work through the changing clientele. For these reasons, material collected from the insurance sector can provide invaluable information on how occupational mental health has been understood within a core area of the private sector that has been subject to various economic, organizational and technological transitions and how the changes have been reflected in the descriptions of employees' mental vulnerability.

In our archival study,[1] we analysed the history of the framing and understanding of mental health issues in the Finnish insurance sector during the period from the mid-1950s to the mid-2010s (Kuokkanen et al, 2020). We examined how the views, arguments and opinions about psychological wellbeing and the status of mental health have changed over time, and who was seen to be responsible for mental health at work. We also analysed whether the processes such as intensification and individualization impacted the views related to employee vulnerability.

Our empirical data consisted of articles from *Kenttämies* and *Pasma*, the two company magazines of a large Finnish insurance company, Pohjola, from 1955 to 2007, and *Vakuutusväki*, the magazine of the trade union of Finnish insurance workers, from 1955 to 2014. Trade union magazines contribute towards constructing professional identities and advocate for the political and economic interests of professional groups (Turtiainen et al, 2018). Company magazines are published by the employer and the final control over the media is in the hands of the employer. However, Pohjola's company magazines also published a great deal of material written by employees. The articles in these magazines offered information on when mental health issues emerged in the discussions, what kinds of concerns were typically reported, the reasons the articles offered for stress and other mental health problems, and how employees were expected to cope with emotional challenges.

[1] An earlier and lengthier version of this section has been published in Kuokkanen, A., Varje, P. and Väänänen, A. (2020). Struggle over employees' psychological well-being: The politization and depolitization of the debate on employee mental health in the Finnish insurance sector. *Management & Organizational History*, 15(3), 252–272. Reprinted by permission of Informa UK Limited, trading as Taylor & Francis Group, www.tandfonline.com. I would like to thank the publisher and the other authors for the permission to republish.

First, our analyses of trade union and company magazines in the 1950s and 1960s showed that only occasional articles referred to work-related mental pressure or mental health. In comparison to the company magazines, the trade union magazine brought up the subject of psychological strain and related mental health problems more frequently. The more critical attitude towards mental pressures in the trade union magazine highlights the differences between the company magazine and the labour union magazine. Many work-related problems were discussed in a more thorough manner in the trade union magazine, while the company magazine could portray the same problems as minor annoyances. However, overall, the topic of mental health appeared strikingly seldom in both magazines when compared to the following decades. Work was presented as a benefit, sometimes even a source of joy, and in a harmonious manner in all magazines. This harmonious image of employer–employee relations is depicted in a quotation from an article reporting a dinner that was organized to celebrate the financial statement of Pohjola in 1965:

> An ant is the symbol of diligence. Our CEO compared us, Pohjola's builders of last year's anthill, to this industrious little worker. ... Awareness of the fact that, guided by skilful management, we can be 'ants', motivates us all to continuously carry out our work more efficiently to offer the best possible customer service. (*Kenttämies*, 3/ 1965, 50)

In the publications of both employees and employers the toning down of criticism and problems was a typical approach. The texts reflect the paternalistic business tradition that has been dominant for a long time. It can be interpreted that the social ethos of the era and the conventions of unconditional paternalistic power were reflected in how grievances were talked about and at the same time prevented the public treatment of grievances, which is common today (Kantola, 2014). The employees were frequently described as subordinates in relation to managers – almost like children – who did not challenge the management. Any criticism that made it into the articles was often disguised as humour. The legitimacy of this kind of management style that is typical of articles of this era rested on the assumption that because the employer had achieved wealth through the work of the employees, he should take care of the employees' needs (Barley and Kunda, 1992: 365–368).

During the 1970s and 1980s, the number of articles discussing mental health problems started to increase, first in the trade union magazine and later in the company magazines. Among the several stressors and mental health risks identified in the articles from the mid-1970s onwards were organizational reformations, workplace rationalization, the introduction of information technology, company mergers, the flood of information, the growing array of insurances to sell and become experts in, the increasing complexity of a clerk's work, growing time pressure, and the new requirements of customer work. Overall, the period marked a considerable turn towards psychological concerns and emotional burdens of employees.

Various mental problems were reported more frequently in the trade union magazine than in the company magazines. The titles reflected growing concern for the psyche of employees: 'The painful problem of the insurance sector – mental health breaks down' (*Vakuutusväki*, 4/1982, 7), 'Insurance company demands too much – a human being is not a machine' (*Vakuutusväki*, 2/1983, 11) and 'We can no longer cope' (*Vakuutusväki*, 9/1985, 4). Stories of mental ill-health were often told by exhausted workers. It was increasingly claimed that employees' mental health problems and psychosocial risk factors did not receive enough attention in the companies. At the beginning of 1980, the trade union released a research report according to which the employees of the insurance sector suffered more mental problems than other workers in Finland. It was claimed that 29 per cent of women who retired before the official retirement age did so because of mental health problems (*Vakuutusväki*, 4/1982, 7).

Discussion on work stress started in *Vakuutusväki* in the latter half of the 1980s and remained a frequent topic until the end of the research period. Psychosocial risks also became a typical label for various challenges emerging at work in the latter half of the 1980s. This meant a new way of structuring workplaces and an effort to more rationally take over a wide range of working conditions that were not seen as part of the official domain in the past (see also Kivistö et al, 2014).

The growing discontent of employees and the tendency to raise mental health challenges can be seen to reflect a change in employees' attitudes and norms towards work and work organization. Discontent with work was indicated in many articles of the 1980s. For instance, the following quote shows how work was now presented more often as something problematic in a person's life. This discourse was completely different compared to the harmonious and untroubled image of work presented in the articles of 1955–1969. 'Several types of changes wear [the employee] out both physically and emotionally. Anxiety and tension increase. Well-being dissolves. People do not trust continuity and cannot predict the future. Insecurity increases. Chronic angst, fatigue and overreactions occur' (*Pasma*, 4/1989, 4).

The financial and insurance sector was severely affected by the post-1970s financial deregulation and the transition from the 'stakeholder' to the 'shareholder' model of corporate governance (Lazonick and O'Sullivan, 2000). The 1970s also saw the beginning of the development of managerialism, that is, the expansion of the area of management, where more and more new organizational aspects were intended to be included in the scope of rational management. At the same time, there were more restructurings of companies, aiming to make operations more efficient and increase production (Ahtokari, 1992: 106–107). In the insurance sector, several reorganizations and mergers took place since the 1980s in Finland (Voutilainen, 2005: 333).

The Scandinavian tradition of quality of work was heavily influenced by the social democratic spirit of industrial democracy and it was manifested in several discussions and projects intending to reduce workers' stress and psychologically inhumane work conditions (Väänänen et al, 2012). The trade union movement was one of the engines of change: it had an integral role in promoting the ideology of quality of work and wellbeing. Since the 1970s, union density was high and reached its peak in the 1990s, when as many as 85 per cent of Finnish workers belonged to a trade union (Hannikainen and Heikkinen, 2006: 174–175). Driven by trade unionism, politics and the media, reformist ideas about work and the necessity of its quality gradually enhanced the possibilities for discussing and addressing topics related to employees' mental wellbeing and subjective experiences, both ideologically, institutionally and discursively. In other words, a new space opened as the society and labour market began to see the employee and the work community as an important part of productivity and organizations' ability to renew themselves. Thus, it is evident that a new sensitivity to the recognition of individuals' mental malaise and an emphasis on psychological wellbeing was created at the same time. In this development, the trade union movement and occupational debates played their own important roles.

At the same time, one of the long-term impacts in work that increasingly sought to solve the challenge of mental vulnerability was the slow revolution in the ideas about employee agency. This change was manifested, for instance, in the new psychological dimensions of occupational safety and the expanded concept of work ability in the 1980s and 1990s (Forma, 2023).

The positive economic boom turned into a sharp decline in the early 1990s in the Finnish economy. Hundreds of thousands of people lost their jobs and unemployment was at a record high (Hannikainen and Heikkinen, 2006). The extensive redundancies also affected the insurance sector. The articles in the magazines of both Pohjola and the trade union indicated that the economic situation was reflected in the employees' wellbeing. Employees were worried about losing their jobs and their future employment. According to many articles, the employees who were not made redundant felt that they were expected to work harder than before, as the same workload was distributed among fewer employees.

Interestingly, our materials from the 1990s imply a beginning of a new period in the mental health discussion in the insurance sector. The period was characterized by an approach that emphasized the employees' own responsibility over their mental wellbeing. Stress management and the ability to regulate one's workload became common themes in both the company and the trade union magazines. Both magazines contained frequent reviews of stress release cassettes and self-help books. Sports, such as yoga, were also described as a means of recovery.

Our materials suggest that the increased national and international competition and market cycles since the 1970s changed the employee's position in the insurance sector. Even though international competition did not dramatically affect the Finnish insurance sector at the end of the 1900s, the rhetoric of competitiveness and needs for increasing efficacy entered the vocabularies and strategies of organizations and of the sector (see Kantola, 2002). Employees were increasingly seen as a replaceable resource for the company. According to employee interviews in the magazines, this also seemed to affect the employees' sense of security, weakening their trust in their employer and resulted in increasing expressions of anxiety. The growing competition between employees was described as eroding the solidarity of the previous decades and making employees more careful about disclosing their difficulties at work. The following extract from our data illustrates this change: 'You cannot do this work if you act with too much solidarity. We have tight objectives, and solidarity can lead to an inability to reach targets, a caution, and a dismissal' (*Vakuutusväki*, 1/2001, 14).

The period between the early 1990s and the early 2010s was marked by a significant transition to individualistic tones in arguments. The political collectivism of the previous period faded. There were fewer discussions on the problems in the organization of work that erode mental health. Instead, the articles reflect how employees were increasingly expected to analyse and assess themselves through psychological concepts and strive towards self-actualization. Rather surprisingly, the trade union magazine fully embraced this new rhetoric and adopted a role in training employees to be competitive individuals.

Overall, our results can be interpreted from the perspective of the social history of market economy and ideologies. The era from the 1940s to the 1960s was dominated by an emphasis on patriotism, national unanimity and the moral duties of the individual. Between the 1960s and the 1980s, these values were substituted by a strong faith in planning, scientific knowledge and collective negotiations. In the 1960s and 1970s, significant economic growth enabled the construction of the welfare state, and the labour unions gained unprecedented political power (Bergholm, 2009). From the 1980s onwards, the emphasis shifted towards market- and competition-friendly individualistic approaches and ideologies (Alasuutari, 1996; Kantola, 2014). Globalization, economic deregulation and the deep recession of the early 1990s impacted the labour market (Siltala, 2007; Bergholm and Bieler, 2013). The transition was economic, technological and cultural. Especially because of the severe economic recession of the 1990s, efficiency requirements increased as fewer people had to produce more services and goods. Digital devices required new skills and made the interaction between the customer and the insurance worker more technology-mediated.

Our findings also indicate that the manifestations of mental vulnerabilities are shaped by organizational and ideological changes in the insurance sector. In the 1950s and 1960s, the organizational culture characterized by paternalistic management did not encourage treating challenges officially at the workplace, and employees did not raise these problems either. This was in line with pathological views dominating public understanding of mental health at the time. Occupational health was pretty much linked to physiological complaints, whereas issues concerning subjective health or emotional challenges were not framed as occupational health concerns by employees, union representatives or health professionals. The period between the 1960s and the 1980s was characterized by many social changes, and the old tradition of paternalism was quietly buried. According to our analysis, the growth in the discussion on mental health seems to have reflected the problematization of an idealized image of work and the former, ostensibly unchallenged, distribution of power within insurance companies. It is evident that changes in the organizational culture as well as the overall broadening of the concept of health played a role in identifying mental health problems as an occupational health risk in the insurance sector.

The democratization of Finnish society and organizations challenged the employees' role as the subjects of the employers' power. Employees were granted a wider and more active role. One outcome of this was that employees were able to express their subjective views more openly and address the sources of occupational distress. Mental health entered the field of occupational health in the form of the psychological wellbeing and mental work ability. The psychosocial work environment was identified as a source of potential mental strain. Subjective dimensions linked to workers' emotional processes and subjective feelings such as work-related wellbeing, work ability and burnout gained wide popularity in the discussions. From the 1990s onwards, the ethos of mental health care came into the spotlight with a culture of psychological self-care and an employee ideal that emphasized flexibility.

Richard Sennett (1998) has claimed that the 'flexible stage' in capitalism, generated by the globalization of labour and capital flows have created a new dialectic of 'flexibility and indifference'. In this permanence-averse culture, the individual needs to keep a strategic distance from others and strive to be flexible in changing conditions that require constant adaptation. Our study illustrates how the change started to call for a social character with a mental health repertoire including discursive, emotional and social capacities of mobilization and adequate psychological functions. It can be thought that the change in work culture has contributed to the creation of a workforce that uses mental health concepts, as the entrepreneur-like character does not seek refuge in a long-term work community but tries to manage on its own, navigating forward using, for example, occupational healthcare.

Echoing the arguments of Ehrenberg (2010, 2017) and others (for example, Honneth, 2004), the problems of social life and work were increasingly seen from the self-structuring perspective of autonomous individuals. Unlike in the 1960s and 1970s, since the early 2000s, social and emotional problems of work and other areas of life were increasingly channelled towards medical and psychological arenas.

The analysis of the occupational debates of the insurance sector indicates that the recent crisis in mental health did not principally evolve during the recent years or even the 21st century. Instead, the socio-cultural emergence of mental health problems among insurance workers gradually developed over a lengthy period of several decades during which new generations of workers started to work and perceive grievances in their work and understand their mental health in a new manner. The emergence of mental vulnerability demanded various changes in the population (for example, values, education), organizations (for example, power structures, leadership), knowledge/ service structure (for example, classification, treatment) and work ability (for example, skills, demands).

To conclude, the rise of mental health challenges in the insurance sector illustrates how mental vulnerabilities we identify today in various business sectors cannot be understood in a comprehensive way by looking at current work conditions and demands caused by the economy. It is important to capture parallel economic and cultural mechanisms fuelling the change. New employee ideals and work ability requirements were far easier to achieve with good mental health but at the same time good social and emotional capabilities also needed fixing in the culture impregnated by productivity demands, customer satisfaction guidelines and wellness norms. Among both less resourceful and more resourceful employees, the challenge of mental vulnerability evolved as an unintentional outcome. This is connected to the fact that the employee's social character was increasingly transformed into an actor understood in psychological terms, from whom more activity was expected in maintaining their work and functional capacity. This was visible, for example, in the discussion and reflection related to emotional challenges in the context of occupational wellbeing. Paradoxically, this 'emancipatory shift' also signified a transition of the area of managing structural problems into the areas of healthcare and psychological knowledge.

The transition of the teachers' behavioural structure

This section deals with how the transition towards late modern work was crafted in the public sector, and especially among teachers. Teachers are one of the core occupational groups who have advanced the process of modernization of the society but who have also been impacted by it in many ways. In countries like Finland, a transition from rural to urban environments after the Second World War has considerably influenced teachers' work as well as the communities in which they work and the kind of school culture they face daily. Therefore, the documents describing teachers' work and work-related challenges over a long course of time provide an intriguing material for the analysis of work, mental health issues as well as the role of social behaviour and work-related demands in the change of the social structure.

We carried out an archival research,[2] in which we analysed the change in the work of teachers and in the discussion of representatives of the profession from the end of the 1930s to the beginning of the 2010s. In the first study on teachers (Anttila and Väänänen, 2013), we analysed articles that were published in the Finnish elementary schoolteachers' weekly professional journal *Opettajain Lehti* (hereafter also referred to as the *Teachers' Journal*, TJ) from the period 1937–1939 and 1948–1950. At the time this was the leading professional journal of Finnish elementary schoolteachers and was owned by the Finnish elementary schoolteachers' national association. We focused on the informal articles, or causeries, that were regularly published in the *Teachers' Journal*. In these articles, several regular writers discussed schoolteachers' everyday problems and experiences on a more personal level than was customary in the more 'serious' articles and editorials in the journal.

Between the 1930s and the early 1950s most of the schools in Finland were in the countryside. The teachers had to keep peace in the schools, and this was based on traditional forms of discipline and the authority of the teachers. Teachers had an important role as front-runners of society, and they had an established social position in the social structure of the community. Finland was on its way to becoming a modern, urbanized nation, while retaining

[2] Earlier and more detailed analyses on this topic have been published in three articles: Anttila, E. and Väänänen, A. (2013). Rural schoolteachers and the pressures of community life: Local and cosmopolitan coping strategies in mid-twentieth-century Finland. *History of Education*, 42(2), 182–203. Reprinted by permission of Informa UK Limited, trading as Taylor & Francis Group, www.tandfonline.com; Anttila, E. and Väänänen, A. (2015). From authority figure to emotion worker: Attitudes towards school discipline in Finnish schoolteachers' journals from the 1950s to the 1980s. *Pedagogy, Culture & Society*, 23(4), 555–574. Copyright © 2015 Pedagogy, Culture & Society, reprinted by permission of Informa UK Limited, trading as Taylor & Francis Group, www.tandfonline.com on behalf of Pedagogy, Culture & Society; and Anttila, E., Turtiainen, J., Varje, P. and Väänänen, A. (2018). Emotional labour in a school of individuals. *Pedagogy, Culture & Society*, 26(2), 215–231. Copyright © 2017 Pedagogy, Culture & Society, reprinted by permission of Informa UK Limited, trading as Taylor & Francis Group, www.tandfonline.com on behalf of Pedagogy, Culture & Society. I would like to thank the publishers and the other authors for the permission to republish.

many of the characteristics of its earlier way of life, such as the importance of the agricultural sector and the strength of local rural communities. The transitional nature of the era was clearly visible in the situation of rural elementary schoolteachers, who by that time had established themselves as important agents in the national modernization project.

When analysing the material, we found that one of the most widely discussed topics was the social pressures and strains that were related to the rural schoolteachers' relationships with their local community, along with the different coping strategies that writers recommended to colleagues who suffered from similar problems. To deal with the pressures of their public position, schoolteachers resorted to different coping strategies which we named 'localistic' and 'cosmopolitan', following Robert K. Merton's (1968) analytical categories. The two strategies had very different implications on the way schoolteachers were orientated towards their local community. The first, the 'localistic strategy', aimed at reducing teachers' social pressures through adaptation and conformity. It required that the teachers adapt their attitudes and behaviours to the demands of community life and strive to make themselves more skilled players in the social field of the local community.

One of the frequent commentators in the *Teachers' Journal* in the late 1930s stressed that isolating oneself from the social life of the community was not a viable option for rural schoolteachers, because this was tantamount to admitting one's failure in the profession. Her advice to teachers who suffered from shyness or social fears was not to give in to these inclinations, but to consciously build their character to become better equipped for the demands of their job:

> [T]here is no other way but to adopt a sterner self-discipline and strive to free oneself from character flaws which may originate from excessive inborn modesty or shyness, as well as from pride. A schoolteacher is, especially here in the countryside, a public person and therefore must cultivate his/her character to endure the obligations and … stresses that his/her position entails. One must learn how to live as a human being among human beings. And to learn that skill, one must often go through a rough school. (Päre Tuikkunen, 'Pelkoa', TJ, 5/1938, 124)

In addition to pro-social character traits, rural schoolteachers needed to have sufficient social tact, foresight and caution in order to survive in their position.

The second strategy, the 'cosmopolitan strategy', in turn, represented a more individualistic and outward-looking approach. It was manifested in teachers' efforts to insulate themselves from the social pressures of community life and to seek personal fulfilment outside the local community. By the mid-20th century, the processes of modernization had already gained a strong influence in the Finnish countryside, connecting the local rural communities ever tighter to the networks and institutions of national society. This allowed the rural teachers to seek a more individualized and specialized professional role, which emphasized the separation of the teacher's private and public roles and confined the latter more clearly to the sphere of the school institution. In terms of psychological challenges, the traditional social role based on authority and the relationship with the local community played a considerable role at work: authority buffered against stresses and the mental strain caused by the social community. However, at this historical point, occupational difficulties were not discussed from the perspective of mental health.

In the next stage of our analyses (Anttila and Väänänen, 2015), we continued analysing the discussions in Teachers' Journal at three points of time: in 1959–1960, 1969–1970 and 1979–1980. In analysing the data, we employed a similar approach to that used by Cas Wouters (Wouters, 1986, 1992, 2007) in his studies on the informalization of social manners during the 20th century. By analysing changes in instructions and etiquette he detected a long-term transition towards less hierarchical forms of social interaction and loosening of tight codes of emotional expression. In our analysis, we compared articles that appeared in professional magazines in different time periods to examine changes that occurred in Finnish schoolteachers' attitudes and everyday teaching methods towards their pupils. We viewed what kind of attitudes and behaviours were becoming unpopular, and what kind of advice teachers were given in dealing with their professional problems. We also observed how the school culture has changed, and monitored the contradictions caused by the reforms and the changing social values. This analytical lens also enabled us to study how these changes influenced the everyday social behaviour and how norms of behaviour related to mental health gradually began to change and gain new meanings in the work of teachers.

The materials reflected how the attitudes towards organizing of schoolwork, social relations and emotional atmosphere in a classroom changed in Finnish schoolteachers' professional discussions between the late 1950s and the early 1980s. At the beginning of the period, the discussion was dominated by conservative views, which saw the increasing unruliness of youths as a serious problem that should be firmly opposed by teachers and the rest of society. Traditional Christian and patriotic values were also to be restored to their former glory. One eminent public figure who advocated such an approach was Professor Edwin Linkomies, a famous academic and a former wartime prime minister of Finland:

> The only way to make this worrying situation better is that parents and teachers alike take a firm grip of the malady. Parents must restore their authority over the young, and teachers must take tough measures to uphold discipline in classrooms and in schools … establishing a firm

grip on youths is essential for the future of our nation. Society must stop pampering youths, because this is harmful even for the youths themselves. (TJ, 49/1959, 4)

However, over the following years, the social climate in Finland became more favourable to progressive and democratic views, and this also reverberated in the teachers' professional discussions. At the turn of the 1970s, hard-line conservative opposition had already given way to views that promoted a more democratic and permissive school culture. The democratic ideals that were characteristic of the reformist period are visible in the following citation, which is an extract from a speech by the then Minister of Education Johannes Virolainen, published in the *Teachers' Journal* in December 1969: 'The Finnish school system has been criticized for its authoritarian spirit. A modern society demands abilities from its citizens which can only be learned in a democratic school. Teaching methods must be remodelled in such a way that they foster the pupils' activeness and their readiness for co-operation' (TJ, 49/1969, 6).

The uncooperative attitude of pupils was an obvious problem in a democratic school, in which the teacher's leadership position was dependent on the pupils' willingness to co-operate. As was pictured by Mirja Pirhonen in the *Teachers' Journal* in 1980, dealing with such pupils in a non-authoritarian way could really test the teacher's emotion management skills:

Through bullying, these children try to lure their classmates into joining their rampaging, and regrettably often succeed in this. As a result, the teacher becomes angry and frustrated. What to do? Teachers should really focus on the situation. They should make use of every available opportunity in which they can express positive feelings towards the [bullying] child. They should also avoid any unnecessary displays of authority that might aggravate the situation further. (TJ, 33/1980, 37)

While the teacher was obliged by legal and professional codes to treat pupils with courtesy and respect in all situations, the pupils had no similar obligations towards the teacher. The quote reveals the same kind of imbalance of mutual obligations and responsibilities which has also been observed in other studies that discuss the problems of modern service work (Bolton and Boyd, 2003; Hochschild, 2003 [1983]: 95–114; Virkki, 2008). This imbalance based on interaction and customer ideology can be seen as a significant change that fuelled various stress experiences that were reported in professional discussions.

By the turn of the 1980s, a progressive view that emphasized respect for the individuality of pupils had become an almost self-evident starting point for discussions on discipline-related problems in schools. Our third period of analysis consisted of articles that were published in the *Teachers' Journal* in

1979–1981, 1989–1991, 1999–2001 and 2009–2011 (Anttila et al, 2018). The emotional demands that the student-centred approach imposed on teachers were considerable according to our material. It required of them a very considerate attitude towards the individual developmental needs and difficulties of children, as well as a readiness to accept a leadership role in the classroom that was much less absolute than it had been in the traditional school (Launonen, 2000: 263–267; Anttila and Väänänen, 2015). In the discussions the difficulty of this challenge was admitted even by those commentators who fully endorsed the ideals of the student-centred school. However, at the same time they emphasized that emotional work demands had to be accepted as an integral part of the teacher's role, as a kind of inevitable price for upholding a democratic school culture that attends to the students' individual needs.

However, the emotional stress involved in student-centred teaching evoked considerable criticism from teachers. These varying attitudes were reflected in the proposed solutions to the problem of teacher stress, which ranged from improving teachers' emotional proficiency to decreasing the amount of emotional work among teachers. Overall, the findings indicate the importance of teachers' emotional demands in upholding the modern individualistic culture. In stark contrast to the earlier conservative views, the writers of the *Teachers' Journal* viewed the teacher as a modern emotion worker who maintained order by carefully managing the emotional atmosphere in the classroom.

The transition was intimately related to the general social change that promoted individualism and social equality in the post-Second World War era. This process eroded the hierarchical social structures in the society and traditional values that had formerly supported the teacher's authoritative position in the classroom. This put great demands on schoolteachers' self-control and emotional management skills, thereby impelling them to adopt an emotionally sensitive approach towards their work (for example, Hargreaves, 1998; Labaree, 2000; Zembylas, 2006).

When viewed from Cas Wouters' (2007) perspective, the new emotional demands of schoolteachers' work can be interpreted as a manifestation of the typical demands that the new age of informal relations makes on individual self-control (cf Wouters, 2007). However, according to our study, the occupational demands of the schoolteachers' work cannot be explained by general cultural change alone; one also needs to consider the changes that have occurred in the specific role that schoolteachers fulfil in modern societies. Whereas in earlier times the schoolteachers' mission was to instil obedience and respect for authorities, in the late 20th century their mission changed to nurturing the individuality and personal growth of their pupils (Simola, 1998; Carlgren et al, 2006). This new role involved human relations work where teachers as emotion workers are required to control their emotions in a much greater way than the pupils (Hochschild, 2003 [1983]; Bolton, 2005: 45–65). In this way, the long-term analysis of teachers' work shows how the discussion on the emotional demands broadened and needs for professional psychosocial support emerged as everyday emotional management gained a new role in teachers' work.

The transition of demands, expectations and norms related to teachers' work illustrates how the modernization of work and culture impacted the status and social behaviour of teachers. As the culture stressing civilized equal interactions and self-management advanced, numerous professionals in addition to teachers had to develop new strategies to cope with the demands caused by individualistic needs and aspirations. It can be interpreted that as Finnish society entered the 'phase of emancipation and resistance' (Wouters, 2007: 184–191) the formality of interactions diminished and the ideology of equality began to gain ground in the 1960s and 1970s. The period was characterized by the upward mobility of large social groups, by the rise of many kinds of social emancipation movements, and by generally positive expectations of the future (Tilly, 2004). The period also witnessed a radical change in the way people understood the meaning of subjective rights. Ironically, this also advanced the development of an expanding mental health concept in the context of work.

The end of the century was characterized by a strengthening of demands related to individualism. Demanding students and active patients are typical examples of pressures of work that are connected to the rise of a new individualistic culture. In the case of teachers, new tasks required considerable psychological understanding of the individual needs and difficulties of pupils, as well as an ability to sense the emotional atmosphere in the classroom and to flexibly adjust their own actions according to the demands of the current situation (Hargreaves, 1998; Labaree, 2000; Zembylas, 2006). In the new professional discussions stress management, work counselling, psychologist consultations and other individual solutions were increasingly discussed. The 'emancipation of emotions' in terms of mental vulnerability were also manifested in the activization of mental health institutions and services. At the same time, the activity of communities suffering from vulnerability, non-government organization activism and the overall politization of mental health took place from the 1990s onwards in many countries (McLaughlin, 2011). As public and formal 'knowing mental health' advanced, more social positions referring to the vulnerability of the psyche were observable and reported.

The long-term occupational and social changes have considerably affected the challenges encountered at work, the ways we view ourselves as workers, the tools of emotional management we use, and the ways we possibly cope with psychological strains encountered at work. The changes also influenced how organizations intended to solve social problems, and how healthcare frames mental health challenges. Hence, the societal and cultural transitions penetrate our personal standards, coping strategies and behavioural options as workers. As the *Teachers' Journal* and other similar materials exemplify, they are expressed in very diverse ways in conversations produced at different times. The professional material also increases the understanding of how general cultural and specific professional development are intertwined in unique ways in the historical descriptions of each profession and ultimately also frames the area of activity defined as occupational health and mental health.

Social work as a form of emotional management

The social sector and social sector occupations have vigorously grown over the past decades in Western countries. This sector differs from the insurance sector and education in terms of purpose of work, customer base, work-related resources and work culture. Employees of social sector have been repeatedly identified as one of the risk groups in terms of mental ill-health (Buscariolli et al, 2018; Kokkinen et al, 2019). Anxiety, depression and burnout are frequently associated with social sector jobs. The social workers' occupation and descriptions by the social workers themselves are likely to provide highly important information on the experiences and interpretations of people working in human service work in the public sector as well as understanding the grassroots level impacts of the transition of the social sector. From the perspective of mental vulnerability, it is important to analyse how the occupational discussions dealing with the nature of work, emotional challenges, employee ideals and forms of work disability have changed in social work as societies have moved from the building of welfare societies to matured modernity. Analysing the descriptions of social workers can produce a new kind of understanding of mental health as a part of a changing society.

In our archival study (Turtiainen et al, 2018, 2022),[3] we investigated social workers' emotional organization of work, with a particular emphasis on how the underlying historical and structural aspects impacted and redefined the emotional labour processes of social work in the latter part of 1900s and the early 2000s, and how the transitions have influenced the ways mental health is positioned and discussed within the sector. The analysis of our

---

[3] Earlier and lengthier versions of this section have been published in two articles: Turtiainen, J., Anttila, E. and Väänänen, A. (2022). Social work, emotion management and the transformation of the welfare state. *Journal of Social Work*, 22(1), 68–86; and Turtiainen, J., Väänänen, A. and Varje, P. (2018). The pressure of objectives and reality: Social workers' perceptions of their occupational complexities in a trade journal in 1958–1999. *Qualitative Social Work*, 17(6), 849–864. Copyright © 2018 by (The Authors) Reprinted by Permission of SAGE Publications. I would like to thank the publishers and the other authors for the permission to republish.

study is based on written contributions by social workers published in their official trade journal, *Social Worker* (SW), from 1955 to 2009. As is typical in union publications, the employees and their representatives pay attention to wages and the status of the work, working conditions and an affirmation of professional identity. However, they also discuss and debate the burdensome aspects of work, the exigencies of interactive jobs and work exhaustion.

The historical roots of social work derive from the pre-war charitable and voluntary welfare organization. The role of the social worker was patronizing and controlling in relation to the clients suffering from poverty in the 1940s and 1950s (Satka, 1994, 1995). From the perspective of the *Social Worker* journal, the creation of the modern social worker character demanded a symbolic cutting of the historical baggage of charitable and voluntary work, as social work gradually developed as municipally organized wage work in the 1950s and 1960s. Social worker and lecturer Helmi Mäki illustrated the ramifications of the shift in client–social worker relationship in 1964:

> According to general information, in their social worker-client relationships social welfare customers incorporate increasingly personal and emotional needs that need to be clarified as a part of, or the background to their problems. The transition from the rural culture to urban, and the rapid social change, which is also realized in the values and norms, causes anxiety. (SW, 1/1964, 24–35)

The management of psychosocial problems required a new readiness to understand the complex challenges and mechanisms behind individual problems. The advocates of the modernization of social work emphasized an understanding of social and psychological problems and the importance of increasing the social worker's professional capabilities. It seems evident that many of the analysed sources from the 1950s and 1960s describe something very similar to what was much later named emotion work.

The rapid societal change and urbanization also offered social workers new opportunities to establish their professional position in the modernizing society. The organization of social workers and trade unionism involved the rise of public sector workers' unionism in the 1970s. As an indication of this, the membership of the social workers' association in 1972 amounted to 1,200 and by 1976 the rate had increased to 3,000 and the union estimated that 80 per cent of all social workers had joined the union. This era initiated the heyday of the welfare state of the mid-1970s and continued through the severe economic recession of the 1990s (Timonen, 2003; Kettunen, 2006). The change in the social sector was transformative. While the welfare costs were 13.6 per cent of the gross national product in 1970, they increased to 25.7 per cent in 1990 (Kosonen, 1998: 110). During the 1990s, there were many cuts for trying to curb rising costs.

Analysing social workers' perceptions of emotion management over several decades enabled us to explore their emotional job requirements, sources of mental strain and perceptions about occupational health. As the contributions were written over a long period of time, we were able to identify the subjects that raised considerable attention among social workers and how the tones and themes changed during the years.

Through the years, the support and supervision of clients' social, psychological and economic problems necessitated social workers' emotional assessment, an empathic predisposition, and the management of interpersonal difficulties. The following extract illustrates this aspect:

> The helper's only tool is their own person, which they try to use to help someone else – the one who needs help. It is important to take a phenomenological stance. This means that the social worker dares to be open and unprejudiced, and comprehensively perceives the distress of another human being. It is important that a worker with empathy and the right orientation settles in the dialogue with the client. (SW, 6/1976, 3)

The emerging vocabulary in the trade journal advocated this development, as the commercial and democratic-sounding term 'client' replaced such stigmatizing words, such as the 'poor' and 'needy', in the 1970s. The emergence of new service work ideology in the social services was connected to the idea of the client's self-determination and an equal relationship with the social worker operating with them. The democratization of the worker–client relationship reinforced the emotional intensity and attentiveness of social work, managing negative emotions, and ultimately the responsibility of social workers for their clients.

During the 1980s, social workers increasingly observed the personal and psychologically demanding aspects of social work. The emotional nature of their work was repeatedly acknowledged as a threat to their health and wellbeing. The catchphrase that a 'social worker's prime tool was their own persona' articulated the problem. Social workers claimed that successful social work required an emotional closeness and intense engagement with the clients' problems and emotional states. One of the first times that 'job burnout' was mentioned in the journal was in 1982 (SW, 6/1982, 3). These issues were explicitly discussed in 1984, when the journal reviewed a survey conducted on social workers in the metropolitan area:

> The mental pressure occurring at work was experienced as a threat to mental health. At work, social workers had to receive anxiety, hopelessness and the fear of disappointment. ... The survey shows that several factors cause a burden to social work, which reduced job

satisfaction. Haste and the excessive number of clients burdened the social workers. Job responsibility and the extent of the work were the most mentally strenuous features. Difficulties in client work and increased bureaucracy may cause feelings of a lack of competence and helplessness. (SW, 14/1984, 4–5)

Based on our material, the concept of emotion management captures the situation and the descriptions in *Social Worker*. Emotional management is a self-regulatory process in which employees control subjective emotional states, emotional dispositions and organizational behaviour (Morris and Feldman, 1997; Bolton, 2005; Lively and Weed, 2014). This behavioural pattern and occupational coping method is guided by both formally and informally internalized professional rules (Hochschild, 1979). Although the professional magazine's descriptions of emotional management stress the structurally determined position of the social worker, employees were seen to have at least some degree of autonomy to self-regulate, adapt and resist the emotional pressures and scripts of work (Bolton, 2005; Ericson and Stacey, 2013). Emotion management was a manifestation of the social worker's contradictory roles as an official or support provider.

In social work, emotion management was largely grounded on the regulations of the welfare policy and practice. The chairman of the union outlines this tension as follows: 'The role of a social worker as a municipal official is problematic. In order to coordinate the official regulations and guidelines and the individual needs and wishes of the client, social workers have to resolve many tricky conflicts of interest' (SW, 6/1985, 4). The articles illustrated how one of the most important skills in social work was the ability to 'read' clients and their emotional states on the basis of their gestures and bodily expressions. In addition to 'reading', social workers utilized expressions such as 'listening' to describe their engagement with their clients. One social worker's quote of a client's opinion of a good social worker in 1987 was in line with this. The quotation stated: 'Of course, one who listens too. Who can ask in a way that you feel that you can easily talk It is a very delicate thing, a matter of subtle nuances. And then that transferring money is not the main thing' (SW, 4/1987, 5).

Numerous social workers objected to the fact that the organization of social work was overtly determined by the administration and that the historical bureaucratic tradition 'still exist(ed) in unwritten procedures' (SW, 5/1986, 8). Though social workers were highly aware that social work was a regulated profession and justified by legal powers, they stated that professionalism did not necessitate facing the client in a bureaucratic or detached manner. To some extent, these notions were the social workers' counteractions to the academic debate on the so-called oppressive and bureaucratic social work of the 1980s (Reamer, 1998; Jones, 2014; Baines and van den Broek, 2016).

These controversies demonstrate the challenges of emotion management in social work and were often present when the psychological burden caused by work was discussed.

Studied materials describe how treating clients with respect and sympathy was an important feature and norm in social work over the decades. These feeling rules highlight how workers' perceptions of their professional identity, and their occupational role were deeply connected to inter- and intra-subjective emotion regulation. The texts they produced describe how their occupational health and psychological wellbeing was closely linked to their encounters with clients and the amount of crucial resources. These notions illustrated social workers' shared understanding of social work as an emotionally demanding human service job, with similarities to nursing and teaching.

A heavy change impacted social work, when a deep economic recession impacted the contents of work through the clients in the first half of the 1990s. In their writings, social workers stated that not only the number of service users had amplified, but the clients suffered from even more serious financial, social and psychological problems. A considerable number of social workers described that their clients had multiple and complex problems, and that excluded people had become even more excluded. At that time, some social workers described their job as 'crisis work'. A social worker summarized the atmosphere: 'Social workers have been forced to become buffers between society and the growing distress of the citizens' (SW, 8/ 1993, 20).

Time pressure and the increased workload left their mark on job discretion and provoked expressions of cynicism and feelings of helplessness in the journal. Social workers' emotional responses became entangled with these extensive quantitative changes, as the following extract illustrates:

> Creating trust in the client and acting as their advocate is essential while calculating the sufficiency of resources. You must be empathetically economical. You have to make individual decisions and at the same browse laws and regulations. We must strive for integrity and at the same time write appropriate reports for the accountant. So, as my supervisor said, this work requires the character of a masochist. (SW, 5/1992, 23)

Many commentators pointed out that welfare cuts and administrative reforms in this period consisted of disconnected objectives, such as organizational accountability and resource limitations, and the simultaneous doctrines of clients' 'activation' and 'empowerment', which were underpinned by the effort towards organizational efficiency and the hope of reducing welfare costs. The previous quote captures the employees' feelings that their professional discretion and emotional regulation were constrained due to economic and administrative causes. Emotional management was very concretely recognized as a condition for success in the profession. A desired organizational behaviour to effectively influence clients in 1996 included the following qualities according to a social worker writing in the journal: 'A smile is a vital part of a social worker's outfit, maintain eye contact with the client all the time when speaking to them, always try to put yourself in the client's position, showing a genuine interest in them, striving to make the client feel good' (SW, 3/1996, 13).

Customer satisfaction and a service-orientation were crucial components of social work. At the same time, the codes and instructions regarding the regulation of emotions indicated that, especially from the 1990s, social workers felt that they were expected to possess the qualifications more commonly found in commercial service industries for better organizational and professional performance and effectiveness. The similarities to 'aesthetic labour' and feminine 'soft skills' (Witz et al, 2003) are striking. Our findings reveal the blurring boundaries of workplace emotions, mainly due to the implementation of efficiency requirements and the reaffirmation of a customer orientation. In a nutshell, the client was portrayed as a 'citizen-consumer', with whom customer service expertise had to be practised.

A focal problem observed in emotion management research, the suppression of genuine reactions and the inconsistency between job requirements and internal feelings, was clearly present in the descriptions of the 1990s and 2000s. The social workers' comments were increasingly overshadowed by psychological burden and the challenging nature of the work.

> According to the textbooks, there are no difficult clients. If a worker wishes to characterize a client as awkward, this sentiment is just a sign of organizational incompetence to meet the client's needs. These lessons come to my mind when a handgun shows up at the door followed by a client. Yes, I recall method lessons and according to them, with threatening clients we should create a relaxing, warm conversation, and aggression should be facilitated in a solution-oriented way. (SW, 7/2002, 8)

The dissonance between the occupation's idealistic guiding principle and real-life encounters felt absurd yet threatening. 'Aggression' was merely an academic term in the textbook of social work, but violence constituted an acute everyday threat to the workers. Similar severe incidents that the social workers brought forth in their contributions also questioned whether occupational safety officials and workplace practices were sufficient to guarantee employees' health and safety at work. In the mid-2000s, according to the national survey, the trade union estimated that 20 per cent of social workers had been subjected to violence in the course of their work.

Our study illustrates how social workers' emotional responses incorporate extra-organizational attributes. In a strongly policy-driven profession, the changes in the welfare state created a feedback loop through economic and social impact, which influenced employees' work and finally their intrapsychic management. This embeds emotional labour in a broader historical context: that of the welfare state, societal reforms and economic turbulence. It is evident that frontline workers gradually became more aware of the emotional cost of emotion management during the research period and recognized its impacts on their psychological wellbeing (Ward and McMurray, 2015).

These results challenge the progressive story of the Nordic welfare regime, exhibiting the 'pain spots' in the execution of welfare policy, and enable us to broadly understand the historical contradictions and complexities which mediate social work. Our analysis of Finnish social work also reflects the ambiguities and tensions found in social workers' experiences identified in other Western countries (Postle, 2002). At the same time, our study indicates how new occupational mental health concerns were related to the transformation of welfare policy and ideology, the rise of white-collar trade unionism, and the change towards emotional management as a fundamental part of work.

These observations mainly correspond with Sharon Bolton's (2005) typology that stresses that in interactional jobs, employees weave their way through different forms of emotional management. In social work, pecuniary, prescriptive, presentational and philanthropic ways of emotional management are stressed. A social worker makes decisions about issues relevant to people's finances, listens, tries to find resources and at the same time is professionally compassionate and philanthropic. Historical analysis indicates how in the first half of the 1990s, large-scale welfare cuts and the retrenchments driven by the economic downturn left their mark on the policy and practice of social work by reducing resources and increasing the severity of the clients' needs. This turn led to a sharp contrast between structural and institutional resources and the actual needs emerging from client work.

There has been a persistent mismatch between the professional ideals held by social workers and the resources provided by the shrinking welfare state. Social workers particularly struggle with the tensions between the occupational norms of philanthropy and strive to help and the shifting welfare regulations and realities. In this regard, social workers have had to shape, reflect and readjust their own emotional labour processes in accordance with public welfare regulations and standards (Postle, 2002; Jones, 2014). At the same time, the work is framed by various interests and social conditions. Working in this field required navigation and psychological means of survival. The expansion of mental health into the area of psychological wellbeing has provided a means of emotional management and a concrete way to deal with demanding feelings privately.

Overall, the grassroots level of the social history of social workers reveals how the profession of social work has been strongly embedded in the needs of a society undergoing modernization. The junctures reflect societal changes, but social workers have also been important agents in creating new vocabularies and conceptualizations in human service occupations and reformulating their occupational experiences. Simultaneously, the debates of social work during a period of 50 years demonstrate how the history of this occupation includes both topics that have continued decade after decade but also various new emerging issues reflecting the ideological climate and economic pressures. Partly surprisingly, in the very early stages of the social workers' discussions we located topics that became influential in sociological studies on work much later (for example, emotional labour).

From the perspective of mental vulnerability, these results show how both occupational history and emerged work demands are present in social work and how the current work culture, which places contradictory demands on workers, can lead to work cynicism and agony. However, the historical material also reveals that mental health approaches and concepts had a considerably low profile in the professional discussions in the 1960s and 1970s. This result illustrates how the challenges of emotional management were dealt with as different concepts and/or how they were not necessarily dealt with at all in the professional discussions. It seems that unionism and collective means to cope with mental strain had a more salient role, especially in the 1970s. The discussions further indicate how mental health concepts and practices related to emotionally challenging work evolved from the 1980s onwards, while the economic turmoil and the overall 'softening' of the discussion on occupational health and work ability towards psycho-emotional concerns opened the debate in the 1990s.

The analysis of social work illustrates how mental health at work is related to the inadequate structural resources to face emotionally burdensome work. In addition to rituals and codes of interaction, broader social hierarchies and the gendered differentiation of the labour market also guide the challenges of managing emotions and their cultural efforts to solve them in social work (Ericson and Staccy, 2013). Interestingly, the history of social work reflects the multi-level entanglement of mental vulnerability with the welfare state, the surge of psychological society and the core challenges and solution models of the female-dominated public social and health sector. To conclude, mental vulnerability became more typical in social work as the problems of work became more intensive, resources for decent work started to decline, and the new paradigms and practices of psychosocial wellbeing/health started to offer acceptable paths to deal with work pressure and the corrosion of professional identity using mental health frameworks.

8

The current dynamics of vulnerability at work

Although history can help to see the layered structure of current work and vulnerability, it is also reasonable to assume that there are specific aspects in current work that affect mental vulnerability, its forms, roles and manifestations. How does our current historical era and way of being and working fuel the escalation of mental health? Which characteristics, challenges and opportunities of work generate the problematization of the psyche? In this chapter, I will particularly focus on knowledge workers, mental health characters among young employees and the difficult challenge of gender in the context of work and mental health.

Tied autonomy and challenged wellbeing among knowledge workers

There are areas of work that did not exist in the 1960s or even the 1980s as we recognize them today. Perhaps the greatest transition has dealt with technology, digitalization and the rise of the information society. This has created a new class of employees: knowledge workers. In the 21st century, knowledge-intensive work has become one of the dominating forms of working. In the EU, the proportion of professionals conducting mostly knowledge-intensive work increased from 13 to 21 per cent and in the Nordic countries from 15 to 30 per cent between 2001 and 2021 (Eurostat, 2022). In this section, I consider whether the analysis of knowledge workers might shed light on the rise and positioning of mental vulnerability in the field of mental health and work. The emergence of new work contents and work structures underlies the need to understand how current mental vulnerabilities may be related to the key features of information-based work and the autonomous character of employees.

Knowledge work is formed from knowledge and other systematically gathered information for application to practical problems. The work benefits greatly from information technology in identifying and solving problems (for example, Alvesson, 2001; Mazmanian et al, 2013). For the most part, knowledge work is done by highly trained professionals working in upper white-collar jobs. Knowledge workers have been accustomed to arranging their own work and schedules themselves (for example, Hellgren et al, 2008a, 2008b). Knowledge work is typically done in networks and projects and requires specialized expertise from various workers, whose tasks are based on mutual interdependencies.

Our interview study[1] consisted of Finnish knowledge employees who worked in knowledge-intensive jobs in Finland in the mid-2010s (Toivanen et al, 2016; Väänänen et al, 2016, 2020). They represented different expert occupations, such as research, communication, public administration and education, and their titles varied considerably. We interviewed planners, specialists, project managers, publicists and educational professionals. We particularly intended to explore the temporal, social and organizational conditions framing work among knowledge professionals and to analyse the implications of these conditions for wellbeing in knowledge work. In addition, we analysed how the work structures and processes differed compared to industrial and clerical work of the earlier periods. From the perspective of mental vulnerability, we asked how knowledge professionals reflected the everyday challenges of their work and occupational health.

We identified different temporal challenges as an essential characteristic of knowledge work and broke them down at different levels. First, on the individual level, the results showed how the interviewees had their own schedules at work that they could not necessarily regulate. In our material, they spoke of how mental work tended to spread out to broader areas (both spatially and temporally) when their minds focused on work-related issues throughout the day and ideas occurred outside the workday. For instance, one of the interviewees noted:

'And all the time, those thoughts are on my mind … if I have to lead a new seminar two weeks from now or training in some new theme that I've been getting ready for a long time, then, of course, it's in my head all the time and I check out my surroundings accordingly and still try to always search for more information. … It is on my mind and my subconscious is also working these things over and they don't disappear.' (Female, non governmental sector)

In this manner, current knowledge work greatly differs from the nature of work done in industrial production, in which enhancing the possibilities

---

[1] Earlier and more detailed analyses on this topic have been published in two articles: Väänänen, A., Toivanen, M. and Lallukka, T. (2020). Lost in autonomy: Temporal structures and their implications for employees' autonomy and well-being among knowledge workers. *Occupational Health Science*, 4(1–2), 83–101; and Toivanen, M., Viljanen, O. and Turpeinen, M. (2016). Aikamatriiseja asiantuntijatyössä [Time matrices in expert work]. *Työelämän tutkimus* [*Working Life Research*], 14(1), 77–94. I would like to thank the publishers and the other authors for the permission to republish.

for even restricted autonomy (for example, breaks, rotation) was an adequate objective because the work itself was fundamentally tied to machinery and assembly lines, with a certain tempo and place. From the perspective of the individual, the role of independence and decision-making power is very different in knowledge work. Knowledge work does not need to be enriched, because it is fundamentally versatile and mentally challenging. The best possible performance at work is often seen to require extensive autonomy and innovativeness produced by it. In applied psychology, the positive consequences of this type of unregulated 'mind-wandering' for creative thinking is emphasized (for example, Baird et al, 2012) and even organizational strategies have started to support innovation and serendipity by creating opportunities for peaceful time for novel discoveries and ideas.

In contrast to these ideals, our interviewees also emphasized how joint meetings and other mutual times that have been agreed on form strong temporal frameworks for one's own schedules. Schedules and meetings are set far in advance, and the days are paced accordingly. The temporal framework and timeline set for project work were often based on a common project plan. Often, creating a common schedule – *time synchrony* – was not easy for our study participants. The more people are involved, the more difficult it is to build a mutual structure. People are busy, "everyone's diary is overbooked" as one interviewee described. The interviewees commented that although colleagues were often physically in the same place at the same time, they were not really present. The challenges arose of how to get people at the same place at the same time and also ensure that they are all mentally aware of what is currently going on. One of the participants explained:

> 'People have experienced or maybe become frustrated, which is certainly true for everyone in today's world, that when you're talking about something, there may be 20 people present and half of them are glued to their own laptops and the rest are focused on their phones, and then you try to explain something that will inspire participation and excite them. And everyone just stares at something and punches a screen.' (Male, private sector)

The preceding quotation also describes the extent to which the social structure has become digitally mediated. Digitalization has supplied specialists with an electronic structure that partly sets the pace of their activity. Digital systems make real-time functioning possible: one's own work can be done even in meetings, but, at the same time, digital systems create new work demands, work interruptions and situations in which several tasks are carried out simultaneously (cf Wajcman and Rose, 2011; Chesley, 2014).

The search for a peaceful time to work is one of the primary characteristics of the individualized attempt for control that marks knowledge work, and it exemplifies the threat to wellbeing, such as irritation, cognitive overload and interruptions, that occurs despite the autonomy of the work.

The resonance of the temporal structures was apparent in our interview material (see also Orlikowski and Yates, 2002). It showed how the social time of knowledge workers is stratified. The so-called interactive time determines personal time, especially if people's own temporal structures have become strongly embedded with others. Knowledge work and organizations have become manifold and interaction at work has become more international and intertwined with many other subjects. At the same time, personal time and opportunities to organize and schedule one's own work have become more limited due to various network dependences and organizational connections.

However, many of the interviewees asserted that the management of their own time "is up to me", emphasizing their own self-reflection and activeness. The acknowledgement of individual competence was viewed as a starting point: people should understand how much is suitable for them; they should know how to put restrictions on their work, and simply make time for their own work. "A sense of self-protection" is needed. This was explained by one of the participants:

> 'But I now also understand that there's never enough time, ever, that that is a utopian situation because, in this type of work, there just aren't any boundaries, you can do as much as you want as fast as you want. So, the only way is to determine yourself what's to be done and when, and talk it over with yourself about where you are, where you can move in safe waters. … And not worry too much about quality, that there just has to be some sort of boundary, that this is the way it is, and that's it.' (Female, non governmental sector)

The interviewees often used such expressions as "I should" and "I have tried". They felt that they were mostly on their own in setting the structures. Management or the boss was "pretty much in the dark about the workers' tasks"; no one had told the experts what they should do, and it was often difficult to determine whether the job was being done or not. On the one hand, the interviews depict the independence of work, one's own responsibility, and, on the other hand, the illusion of autonomy. For many professionals, the control of individualistic work as being autonomous had turned into uncontrolled running to meet a minute-by-minute schedule. Often work time spread past normal working hours, and cognitive pressure easily remained in place. This situation is also reflected in occupational health, as shown in the following quotation:

'[S]ometimes there are weeks when everything piles up and there are impossible schedules and such demands that I have to be ready to deal with. And then in that week there're also all kinds of other needs to take care of, and I have a kind of robot-like feeling. In other words, I'm pulled in all directions. … In the evening I think about everything I need to put reminders about into my phone so that I'll remember to do things the next day. And it may be that, by Friday I've such a feeling that I'm really not able to forget about the week, so I sleep really restlessly. And in the evenings I'm so tired. … There can be some weeks when I'm really exhausted, going from meeting to meeting with a minute-by-minute schedule and thinking about how I can possibly get everything done.' (Female, public sector)

In this way, autonomy, which characterizes knowledge work, left people doing work on their own. The hectic rhythm of work and continuous self-structuring was easily reflected in psychological and somatic wellbeing. In many interviews, the mental load, exhaustion and sleeplessness came up. The feeling of insufficiency was due to social ties, overlapping schedules and choices. A dead end was set by the interface between individual responsibility and complex social ties, so that, along with work results, subjective endurance and navigation was considered to be the responsibility of the individual. Given this, it becomes understandable that autonomous knowledge work can produce both positive (for example, high sense of personal accomplishment, strong motivation, low absenteeism) and negative (for example, limitless stress, burden of decision-making, tenseness) individual and organizational consequences.

To summarize, in today's knowledge work the topic of control and management is quite different than in the period of the industrial regime in the 1960s and 1970s. Networks and temporal dependencies create a situation that we have defined with the concept of 'tied autonomy' (Toivanen et al, 2016; Väänänen and Toivanen, 2018; Väänänen et al, 2020). It is characterized by a high level of individual freedom to make decisions and plan one's work, but also by a high level of temporal interdependency and social ties, because the work process itself is embedded in multiple social and organizational relationships (Väänänen and Toivanen, 2018). In this context, autonomy has a rather illusory nature. Under these historical conditions, new forms of and ways of organizing work generate a different occupational strain environment, in which the subjectivity of the employees experiences continuous demands due to temporal and social structures.

The foundations of current occupational health thinking were developed in the 1960s and 1970s during the era of a strong industrial sector and when rather unchallenging, simple and pre-structured office jobs existed. The initial objective of work and occupational psychology was to make work more decent and develop 'psychosocial resources' to combat poor working conditions (Frankenhaeuser and Gardell, 1976; Gardell, 1976; Hackman and Oldham, 1976). From the perspective of knowledge work it is relevant to ask whether this kind of thinking is still relevant to the current work environment and wellbeing at work. The nature of knowledge work and tied autonomy calls for new thinking about wellbeing at work and work ability, as both the characteristics of work and the cultural essence of the employee have changed. The current heterogeneity of work also makes us think about the extent to which universal models of occupational wellbeing can work, when the development targets are often very different depending on the job and work culture.

The paradoxical nature of autonomy means that psychosocial and organizational factors at work may have distinctive meanings and impacts depending on the social and occupational context. These results show how knowledge professionals rationalize their behaviour, and how they try to cope within the limits of 'tied autonomy'. They also indicate how their core structure of work and life quite considerably differs from the work and life of the generations of the industrial era. The critical tension between autonomy and control has reached a new phase in knowledge work (Andersen et al, 2022). However, the mechanized control coming from outside is not substituted in a sustainable way only by the inner self-control and management.

The illusion of autonomy among knowledge workers illustrates that the combination of cognitively intensive work and the high-level of demands for self-structuring may lead to unwanted psychological consequences. For instance, we found a high prevalence of memory deficits, sleep disturbances, anxiety and symptoms of exhaustion among Finnish knowledge workers (Toivanen et al, 2016). In this way, Alain Ehrenberg's (2010, 2017) analysis of the detrimental impacts of continuous self-structuring seems to capture something relevant in relation to the analysis of knowledge workers' mental vulnerability. This means that also studies on work–related mental health and psychological wellbeing would benefit from the understanding of historical change in self-structuring demands in relation to work and other spheres of life.

Tied autonomy and the structural interdependency of knowledge work is related to the flexible forms of capitalism at the beginning of the 21st century and its socio-cognitive nature. Knowledge workers repeatedly described how time dependencies and larger production cycles created interdependency and various butterfly effects. Our finding reflects the paradoxical situation in which more flexibility at the level of the individual is required in late modernity but simultaneously flexibility on the societal scale may be reduced (Eriksen, 2016: 87). Applying a stress perspective, the cognitive scale expands, and networks are much larger, which creates more interdependency, but our Stone-Age brains are still accustomed to dealing with different types of micro-level challenges. Hence, complexity not only increases vulnerability on the societal level, but it has several emotional and psychological impacts at the individual level. Often employees encounter these tensions in their work when it is supposed to be autonomous and individually organized.

Interestingly, the observations of our interview study are linked to the work by some critical philosophers and social theorists who state that we have moved to the stage of cognitive capitalism (Moulier-Boutang, 2011; see also Braidotti, 2019: 93). Cognitive capitalism means that the production of wealth takes place increasingly through knowledge, through the use of those resources of labour that are defined by cognitive activity (cognitive labour). This new stage of capitalism is characterized by the importance of immaterial elements, deriving directly from employment of the relational, affective and cerebral faculties of human beings. It takes place through a wide variety of new labour processes made possible by the development of digital technologies of communication and intensified forms of networking within this system of production. In this historical stage of capitalism, individualized contractual relations and self-based navigation become more common, which can be seen in many of our interview materials.

This perspective offers an important framework for understanding the connection between the human qualities required in the workplaces and the historical transition of the labour market. The shift in the structure of the 'social behavioural network' influences us and our psychological concerns. Ehrenberg's (2010: 98) claim that today we obey by carrying out tasks instead of obeying orders mechanically seems a relevant argument from the perspective of knowledge workers. Completing tasks leaves more leeway than mechanically following detailed commands. It is not therefore surprising that among knowledge workers in particular there have been numerous discussions about work and professional identities, self, self-management and subjectivity over the past 20 years. Work has increasingly become a platform for completing the task of meaningfulness and personal development.

'Tied autonomy' is experienced within the cultural context of late modern individualistic psychological humanism. From the perspective of population and value changes, there are numerous cultural and institutional changes that are linked to the turn to problematic autonomy: the emergence of individualization, 1960s protest movements, humanization of work, rise of therapeutic culture, feminization of culture, doctrines of wellbeing at work and work psychology, human-centred educational ideals, and human resource management discourses – among others (for example, Julkunen, 2008: 122).

In this way, new demands of the economy and the shift towards new social forms of character and emotional strategies are closely interrelated with mental vulnerability in knowledge work. The social analysis of the nature of knowledge work and psycho-emotional wellbeing provides an important avenue to observe the change in the core structure of occupational health and work ability over the past 30 years. The problem with tied autonomy shows how organizational and socio-structural dimensions are in such an important position in the map of work-related vulnerability. At the same time, it is somewhat ironic that transitions at the level of labour market and culture affecting the fundamental structure of our subjectivity as workers are increasingly dealt with in healthcare using vocabularies of work ability, therapy and treatment. Overall, the parallelism between socio-organizational dependence and heightened autonomy opens up a view of increased expressions of mental vulnerability in certain segments of the population.

Social character formation among young employees

Since the beginning of the 21st century there has been a substantial increase in the number of younger persons with mental health problems entering disability benefit schemes in many EU and Organisation for Economic Co-operation and Development countries (Prins, 2013). For example, the Netherlands, Sweden, Norway and the UK have witnessed an alarming pattern of development. Among young adults, most disability benefit claims are related to mental ill-health in the 2010s (OECD, 2015). In Finland more than 75 per cent of work disability retirements are related to mental disorders among under-35-year-olds, while among the oldest age groups the same share is less than 15 per cent (Laaksonen and Blomgren, 2020). Depression and anxiety-related sickness absences have also increased especially among younger age groups. The most dramatic change was observed among women aged 16–34 whose depression-related episodes increased two-fold and anxiety-related episodes almost five-fold in 2005–2021 (Blomgren and Perhoniemi, 2022).

In one of our qualitative studies, we investigated this complex topic by analysing young adults' structure of mental health and work from the framework of everyday social codes and behavioural options. How do young employees working in different positions and occupations end up with mental-health-related solutions? What kind of behaviours and interpretations could be found concerning the development of mental vulnerabilities? What is the role of work? What else could be hidden behind the problems that appear as psychological work ability challenges? What do young adults themselves think and what ideas and observations do the supervisors and health professionals who work with young people have?

In our interview study (Lehmuskoski et al, 2022),[2] we did not look for risk factors and causal explanations but sought to reach descriptions of

---

[2] An earlier and lengthier version of this section has been published in: Lehmuskoski, K., Väänänen, A., Juvonen-Posti, P. and Mattila-Holappa, P. (2022). Mielenterveyden

the social and material frameworks of activities from which the challenges related to work ability and mental health of young adults in the early 2020s are developing. We gathered the interview material from the municipal sector from the metropolitan area of Helsinki, where employees' mental-health-related problems have considerably increased in line with general development (Sumanen et al, 2020). Most of the interviewees were young adults, both those who had sought help for their mental health symptoms, and those who reported they had not. We also carried out various interviews with occupational healthcare professionals and supervisors. Altogether the wide interview material consisted of 70 interviewees. The study included many municipal occupations where the use of occupational healthcare services is substantial, such as childcare, education, and social and healthcare services, technical support as well as several other occupational sectors within municipalities.

As a general analytical framework, we focused on the forms of social character that are employed and socially shared in the area of work-related mental health among young employees. This approach consciously intends to overcome frameworks and shortcomings of risk-based epidemiological research and variable-based psychosocial research concerning mental health in a work context, often leading to individualistic views on work, health and disability. According to this perspective, mental health is an integral part of our social action and institutional relationships. As described in Chapter 2, the concept of social character forms a meso-level linkage between structural conditions (for example, work conditions, cultural values, medical classifications) and individuals (for example, identity, motives, emotions) (Shilling and Mellor, 2022). By using the social character approach and analysing the overall conditions and possibilities of social behaviour, it is possible to capture how mental vulnerabilities are shaped and formed in certain material and social conditions and in various sub-cultures of young employees. It also helps to understand why mental health has become such a dominant framework in dealing with mundane challenges of life and work.

Altogether, seven social character formulations related to mental health were identified from the interview material. The aim of the typology was not to categorize individuals, but to describe cultural models and typical tensions which fuel the surge of different mental health trajectories among young municipal employees and produce various forms of mental vulnerability.

toimijahahmot: Laadullinen tutkimus nuorista työntekijöistä kuntasektorilla [Social characters of mental health. A qualitative study of young employees in the municipal sector]. *Kuntoutus* [*Rehabilitation*], 45(4), 6–19. I would like to thank the publisher and the other authors for the permission to republish.

The first character detected was a *professional losing their ideals*. This character often works in ethically stressful work, in the profession of early education, teaching or in social and healthcare. The workload per person is meticulously calculated to maximum capacity per person by default and the recruitment problems of the field aggravate the situation at the workplace. The problems with mental health arise mainly because the ideals of the profession are repeatedly crushed by the daily reality at work. This quote from the headteacher of a comprehensive school describes how she views the situation among the younger colleagues in schools: "[T]hey are quite idealistic, so it feels like whoever has created or creates those goals there, it somehow feels like there's not so much a conception of the everyday life and the reality that is going on there in the field" (headteacher, female, born in the 1970s).

Many young interviewees linked to this social character felt that they were in the right line of work, but the mismatch between their ideals and reality could drive them to think about changing to a different profession. The mental health challenges of the *professional losing their ideals* arise from the scarcity of resources and broken promises: the initial function of the job – for example, education or care – is not achievable with the available resources. Due to the structural nature of the problem, it is difficult to find a solution to the emotional problems of this character. In the long run, the unbearable situation easily feeds frustration, anxiety and symptoms of burnout.

The second social character detected in the descriptions of mental health challenges provided by the interviewees was also related to the scarcity of work-related resources. We described this character as a *fragile human professions expert*. This character works in a low-paid, female-dominated industry, typically in homecare or childcare, often in similar workplaces as the *professional losing their ideals*. In addition to an ethically and emotionally charged job, adverse experiences in childhood and/or youth and accumulated difficulties in their personal life in adulthood lead to mental vulnerability. Often occupational health professionals described this type of character as follows:

'[T]hey are wonderful people, who have often gravitated to the field from a place of great interest and a desire to work with children and youth and often want to do it with pleasure. But then they may, unfortunately, have many bruising experiences in life and very difficult things they have had to experience, already in the childhood family and in the school world.' (Psychiatric nurse, female, born in the 1970s)

This social character also tends to search for help for acute anxiety and hopelessness in occupational healthcare. According to the interview materials, the coping strategy often used by this social character is talking about the issues of their emotional and/or personal life in the workplace and this may burden other employees as the collective resources (for example, temporal) for handling emotional problems in the work community are often thin. In the background, the economic situation and other core resources seldom offer a solution to solving problems at work and in other spheres of life. To summarize, the problems of this social character stem from a scarcity of resources and a narrow scope for action, such as loneliness and intergenerational disadvantage. In this way, the mental vulnerability of this social character is strongly linked to the structural challenges arising from the work and other spheres of life that are eventually manifested in the mental challenges treated in occupational healthcare.

As the third mental-health-related character, our interview material contained many descriptions about a subject who was uncertain about their future. According to this narrative, current society and labour market demand a lot and you have to keep up with the pace. The character that we labelled the *risk-aware reflector* not only recognized the potential risks arising from work and the cycles of economy but also stressed the individual effort in anticipating risks and preparing for them in advance:

> 'I feel that even if I already have two … degrees in the background, it is not enough in these days. If you already have a job, then you have to be a bit like multi-skilled. … Thereby, thinking about these sickness absences, not everyone has enough resources to this kind of blasting all the time.' (Exercise advisor, female, born in the 1990s)

This character type is born out of the perceived competitiveness. In the municipal sector, the protagonist often works in a relatively low-paid position, but keeps retraining alongside work, because this character form hopes to see themselves in a better paid job in the future. The problems of the risk-aware reflector surface from both the scarcity and abundance of resources: this character aims to pursue security and continuity in an unstable time, and at the same time, make use of the abundance of resources and opportunities for development. In this way, the worries, fears and despairs of this character are fuelled by the fear of economic recession and changes in work, and this is substituted by the investment in personal growth and self-reflexivity.

The fourth social character identified from our interviews was the *autonomous self-developer*. For this character, autonomy is an ultimate concern that is prioritized above certainty and continuity. They are the independent individuals of the theories describing the late modern period, always looking for new meanings and making progress. Autonomy-seeking and development-orientated social figures usually work in professional positions requiring a higher education. At work, they are burdened by the old-fashioned leadership of the municipal sector, and this can be a reason for them to switch to a different workplace. One of the interviewees notes: "And because of it I'm in an existential crisis about what motivates me in my work, when I feel that in this moment I am not learning very much, so, I'm not developing so to speak" (communications specialist, female, born in the 1990s). This social character emphasizes the importance of listening to oneself and the inferiority of current work in relation to one's own values and ideals. Work needs to fulfil the inner motives of the self. They have often already achieved a lot but are unsure about how to proceed and what choices they should make. For such characters, the need for self-development was also a source of contradiction: missing opportunities was experienced as depressing, yet new opportunities brought exhaustion and anxiety because they often led to multiple options and the need for further auto-reflection and decision-making.

The mental vulnerability of the autonomous self-developer stems from the abundance of options and many desired and real-life projects, the coordinates of which are sought within one's own identity and personal goals. Sickness absences are experienced as temporary flag stops that enable withdrawing from work life and creating a new action strategy. In this manner, new developmental aims, seeking new meaningful contents and the demands of self-integrity are both potential sources of mental satisfaction and vulnerability for this character.

Interestingly, the difference between a traditional working career model and the late modern individualistic life career was often seen in the interviews. In our analysis, we identified a social character who was engaged with traditional protestant values of work. Unlike the two previous agent characters, the agency of the *traditional working morale professional* is framed by normatively binding habits and practices. These character models are typically found in physically taxing professions where work itself is seen as prestigious. The traditional working morale professional does not easily turn to occupational health services when encountered with psychologically burdening situations, but usually intends to cope without professional help by speaking with their close persons and workmates. The following interview extract illustrates these traits:

'So somehow for older people, the working morale is much higher, because then you've grown up [with the idea that] you go to work and get money. And like, in a way that is where you aim to go in life. But it is after all maybe not like that for the young anymore, like everyone wants more somehow. They want that the work is meaningful, and you have a career, and should get more money. Somehow, to be like successful, on a higher level. When before it was somehow quite OK that you were a school cook and you were proud of it.' (Food service respondent-in-charge, female, born in the 1990s)

Because the interviewees evaluate their personal situation in relation to the social appreciation they receive, the traditional working morale professional may feel like decent work is no longer appreciated and the values of the new culture of work do not correspond with their moral compass. This character feels alienated and suffers because of the cultural turn highlighting the importance of emotionally rewarding experiences at work and fulfilling the supreme values of the identity. They also suspect the advantage of medical and psychological approaches in dealing with work–related and personal problems. The dissatisfaction of this character frequently arises from the conflict between one's own values and the ideals of new individualism as well as the lack of social status and economic assets.

One of the mega–trends of the current economy and labour market is related to the importance of cognitive and social know-how in work requirements and ideals. According to our interviews, it seems that the structural dynamics underlying young employees' mental–health–related disabilities could be linked to undetected learning and attention–related problems that present themselves in the demands and complicated environments of workplaces. We named the sixth social character *the underperforming character*. This character type can be hard to detect in occupational healthcare, even if they themselves might have had, for a long time, a suspicion about the cognitive and/or neurological root of their problems. This social character was often recognized in the interviews of occupational health professionals: "Behind these perseverance and ability questions, it seems like a big group are these untreated and undiagnosed learning difficulties from childhood and youth" (occupational health doctor, female, born in the 1960s).

In the interviews, it surfaced that the mental vulnerability of this social character was caused by situations in which striving does not produce visible results, they feel that they are failing, and the individual is labelled lazy or stupid at the workplace. Failures can diminish faith in their opportunities and make the character withdraw from actively orienting their own life. It seems that the transition of work contexts and the efficiency demands of intensified economy do not offer similar positions as earlier welfare society for employees who do not have sufficient resources required in new work marked by interaction, abstract thinking and digital systems. This creates new pressures in the arena of occupational mental health as well as demands for developing new categories and processes of mental work disability.

Finally, in occupational healthcare, there are various descriptions concerning a social character who comes to the practice because of a somatic problem. After investigation, emotional issues and often risky use of substances can be found to be underlying. In these cases, psychological symptoms can be paralysing and demand an urgent psychiatric diagnostic review. As this social character is related to the masculinity and the traditional way of dealing with emotional problems among men, we labelled this character the *silent man*. The occupational health representatives describe this character as someone who is sometimes rewarding to help, but sometimes can render professionals helpless and, in worst case scenarios, very late.

The silent man was often described by the interviewees as a history-less and unchanging social character, against which the progress and need for development of the modern man were often compared. The social models of behaviour that embodied the silent man were seen to be transferred from one generation to another. Therefore, the character of silent man underlies the role of gender in the social order of mental vulnerabilities by indicating how most other social characters associated with current mental health are dominated by behavioural strategies and solution-seeking models traditionally considered feminine.

The results show that there are many challenges stemming from various operational friction points under the mental health category among young employees. Many of them are not mental health problems of individuals, per se, but related to other trajectories or sources of strain that are increasingly intended to be resolved in healthcare. For instance, the social character formations suffering from insufficient work conditions and personal resources (for example, the professional losing their ideals, the fragile human professions expert and the underperforming subject) highlight the considerable importance of the real-life circumstances of work. Often lack of time and qualified substitutes, the increasing flow of demanding clients, pressures of making unethical decisions and other demands of work are everyday life for thousands of municipal workers. At the level of the psyche and the work community, there seems to be concrete shortcomings with some qualities of work that are essential for decent performance and solid wellbeing. Currently these problems are constructed as mental health issues in our cultural and institutional practice through different social characters.

The social characters indicate that, in terms of working capacity, it is one thing to act and build a life from the perspective of an educated middle-class person with several competing life goals, but it is another thing to work in the midst of material poverty and overburdening working conditions. Child- and homecare, social work and nursing assistance are examples of municipal work in which conditions are repeatedly reported as being psychologically and physically burdening and their core problems are not primarily related to autonomous subjectivity or therapeutic culture. Their challenges are palpable. However, I still argue that the identity challenges, problems brought by being oneself and the liberation of emotional expressivity are increasingly recognized and intervene in the occupational sectors of material scarcity as well.

The detected characters seem to be connected to the problematization of material progress, the increasing efficiency requirements and the disillusionment of several segments of workers concerning their prospects. Today, the reality of municipal work done in welfare countries does not seem to be like social reformists hoped at the beginning of the welfare societies 50–60 years ago. Thomas Hylland Eriksen (2016: 74) describes this as the broken promise of unilinear social evolutionism, associated with the erosion of future-reliant prospects and appearance of new limits. From the perspective of mass psychology, it is evident that the trust in ever-developing and future-believing identities has been questioned in Western populations. There is a rise in the number of people in Finland and other welfare countries who are looking for themselves and who are looking for their place in society and labour market but have difficulties in finding a suitable position. This can also be seen resonating in mental health services.

The characters of the *autonomous self-developer* and *risk-aware reflector* represent discursive solutions that have become common in late modern work culture, but also action strategies that are considered culturally rational. This approach could be called self-listening and self-directing morality. The education of the generations born in the 1980s and 1990s was based on the recognition of individual differences and the encouragement of norms that underlined the importance of finding one's individual path in life. They grew up in the atmosphere of psychological humanism. Many currently struggle in work which offers numerous developmental opportunities and requirements in conjunction with unstable future views. Despite expectations of upward social mobility and the general realization of rewarding individual options, life is typically characterized by middle-range compromises and a search for pieces of meaningfulness.

The character of the *risk-aware reflector* crystallizes something essential about our time. It emphasizes the potential danger of falling and a need to strengthen various personal capabilities to guarantee one's position and labour market value. The source of the psychological burden arises from the perceived societal and economic situation as well as the individualistic strategies for coping that stress the importance of risk-awareness and proactivity. In this manner, this character illustrates several qualities that are typical for workers in affluent economies accustomed to evaluating the risks of everyday life and self-labelling their emotional difficulties (Thoits, 1985; Petersen and Wilkinson, 2008). The reflexivity of the character also means that inner motives and self-related objectives are also part of the evaluation process.

The direction must be found by the autonomous and reflexive subject, since the persons themselves have become the source of ethics (Taylor, 1992; Rosa, 2003; Côté, 2019; Fowers et al, 2021: 80). The notion of authenticity stresses commitment to self-values. In this moral framework, one intends to be true to oneself. Reflection can also lead to 'colonising the future', in which case nightmare scenarios that might not happen provoke psychological distress (Saastamoinen, 2006: 142–144). The demand to be able to reflect one's own thinking and the choices made causes mental pressure (Furedi, 2004; Archer, 2012). Reflectivity is also used to outline the direction of action and promote wellbeing. It is possible that this subjectification and psychologization of work ability/disability leads to the increasing observations and discourses of mental vulnerability in occupational health, because reflexivity is accompanied by a need for professional discussion and the evaluation of one's situation. It includes consideration of individual strategic choices and emotion-based reflection of future prospects.

From this perspective, individual symptoms of mental vulnerability in late modern character types are not only determined by excessive demands produced by organization and management but also by problems in fulfilling social expectations and obligations of self-realization (Vannini and Williams, 2009). Work and self-values reach down into the identity of the employees. Failure to realize oneself is not just experienced as a professional failure but also as a personal failure. In this way, being a late modern subject is likely to generate expressions of psychological vulnerability that were less typical in earlier historical periods.

The social transition of the character signifies a possibility and a necessity to mobilize, invest and express one's thoughts. Employees are expected to adopt new approaches, use social skills, show emotional receptiveness, and have the ability to handle mental pressure. The transition towards psychologically toned vulnerabilities is not just transition of risk environments, but mental vulnerability is caused by an unpleasant conflict that arises between the character's (desired) ideals and actual personal positions at work and in other areas of life. The inner conflict between limited opportunities of work and limitless thinkable social character options leads to insecurity about the right direction and continuous need for self-reflection. At the population level the prevalent ideals concerning social character do not match the character forms available in the real-life settings and this creates pressure for psychological work and self-reflection.

The perspective of cultural availability of social character forms is largely ignored in academic literature focusing on the modelling of work environmental and individual characteristics and their combinations. In this context, meanings, ideals and norms employees attach to work, emotions and wellbeing in the historical context remain undetected. To understand the phenomenon labelled as a mental health crisis, it might be relevant to ask how our material and cultural structures of being and becoming social subjects (both at work and outside it) have changed so that we need and call for frameworks like mental health.

Our results on social character forms can be placed amidst wider changes in work and the labour force. When the national *Working Conditions Study* in Finland began in 1977, only 28 per cent of Finnish wage earners felt that the opportunities for self-development at work were good. In 2018, the corresponding number was 45 per cent (Sutela et al, 2019). The occupational structure has changed towards white-collar and professional roles, and this has strongly affected the opportunities to develop oneself at work. Additionally, at the personal level, Finnish wage earners have increasingly seen self-development to be important (in the year 2018, 58 per cent did). Person-related development has become a lot more important than opportunities for career progress for many. The reverse of this long-term trend is that the paradigm of individualistic development can lead to a far-reaching compulsion to develop oneself and feelings of psychological burden. If no boundaries are set for development claims (and the psyche), the growth of development opportunities and quests for further capacities can lead to both new intellectual and technical capital but also unfavourable results for the psyche. Hence, a strong emphasis on oneself without a meaningful societal purpose can produce ever greater experiences of redundancy and meaninglessness (Honneth, 2004).

From the broader rubric of humanization and democratization of work and society, it could be stated that the tendencies and ideals of democratic societies have led to the acknowledgement of workers as thinking subjects and responsible beings. The cultural values of the end of the 20th century and the beginning of the 21st century emphasize equality, attention to individual needs and doing things that are important to oneself. This tendency is likely to be more pronounced among younger generations who have grown up in the culture of the era, stressing individual characteristics and personal life targets instead of class-based, political, religious or other traditional commitments and ethical guidelines (Shilling and Mellor, 2022).

Given this macro-context, it is understandable that psychological vocabularies and therapeutic approaches are felt to be necessary. It is important to find ways to affirm and claim oneself and psychological means are planned to facilitate the delivery of this task. In this cultural mindset subjects increasingly seek answers in professional practices of mental health. Indeed, many of the dynamics of vulnerability manifested in the late modern actor character arise from trying to solve individual life challenges in a morally sustainable way, and the mental health field provides a legitimate platform for this work. Rather than turning to a priest to confess and absolve our sins, modern individuals rely on psychological advice for guidance, comfort and direction (Fejes and Dahlstedt, 2013). From this point of view, the growth of the mental health field and mental health services is not a solution but rather a symptom produced by a long process.

It seems that currently working on emotions and modifying one's psychological state is a much more central part of the formation of work ability and health than before. This tendency has also been influenced by new practices of becoming oneself and social belonging to a work organization (Andersen et al, 2022). From this perspective, the late modern identity is not an outcome of therapeutic culture but being a social and moral character in the 2020s calls for mental vulnerability and working on it. The observed therapeutic needs also provoke disagreements and tensions between generations, because professionals and supervisors of a different generation (mainly born between the 1950s and the early 1980s) reflect upon the challenges of the young mind. Many of them bring out their difficulties to understand the current psychological distress and the increasing need for professional support when looking at the phenomenon from the perspective of their own life history. For instance, among some older generations the development of the psychological/psychiatric filter also raises morally attuned questions about the sensitivity of the younger generation and critical reflection on the current nature of mental health.

These observations tell us something essential about the difference between the current expanded concept of mental health and the meagre concept of mental illness of the past. It also emphasizes the naming of oneself with the concepts of mental health: 'I had a panic attack', 'I got anxious' and 'I got burnt out' in the new landscape (on 'self-labeling', see Thoits, 1985) Psychological and psychiatric paradigms have spread in the attitudes and repertoire of actions, but there are still many alternative perspectives and behavioural strategies among young employees, as our results from the municipal sector occupations indicate.

In our analysis, the 'worker with traditional ethics' and the 'silent man' represent social forms of being a worker that are rooted in the more material and corporeal image of the subjectivity. They stress the fundamental value of the work as a source of income and decent working conditions in the context of delivering one's work tasks. From the historical perspective of occupational health, these social character types recognize the transition of the work and work cultures towards psychological and non-material characteristics, but they prefer a view of occupational health as a traditional arena of workplace hazards and somatic problems. This occupational health view is most evidently manifested in problems caused by the inhalation of asbestos dust, industrial noise, accidents related to dangerous machines and human error or unhealthy ergonomics. Health-eroding aspects of work are seen to be physical, chemical and/or biological, while psycho–emotional characteristics are not integrated in this 'organic' conceptualization of occupational health. The inner tumult and vulnerability of subjectivity are seldom present in this interpretative context.

The 'worker with traditional ethics' and the 'silent man' also indicate that class and occupation specific social norms influence our views on work ability and how it should be (Bourdieu, 1984: 244; Doblytė, 2019). These subjects stressing the codes of physical health and somatic work ability themselves do not identify with therapeutic conceptualizations and narratives. Their relevance is doubted or felt to be distant. This point also calls for an analysis of gendered ways of 'doing mental health' that will be addressed in the next section.

The typology of the mental health characters indicates that the perspective of literate social gradients is over-represented in many critical theories stressing the downsides of individualization. The problems with extended self-autonomy, the continuous need for choice-making and identity projects are indeed sources of increasing mental stress and problematizations, but not for all. Our materials address the fact that young workers coming from different backgrounds and representing different positions employ a wide variety of mental health frameworks and prefer different cultural character forms in their behaviour. Many of them distance themselves from the therapeutic vocabularies and psychological frameworks.

In terms of increasing occupational disabilities these findings provide a window into how the medicalization, psychologization, intensification and other mega-trends are acted upon in daily life settings and how they actualize in the behaviours of young employees occupying different social positions. It seems evident that mental health has become a more common trajectory for increasing number of people representing younger generations, and the character formations of mental vulnerability are fertilized by a large set of medical and psychological frameworks and institutional solution models. Viewed from a distance, the phenomenon appears as a mental health crisis, but upon closer examination, many different paths begin to appear, where cultural differences and the multiple contexts of work are visible. The social upheaval that took place since the 1960s and 1970s seems to have quietly shifted the handling of multiple challenges to the area called mental health. This is clearly reflected in the situation of young working adults in the 2020s.

The gendering of mental vulnerability at work

The World Health Organization, the EU (for example, WHO, 2002; OECD, 2015) and numerous scientific studies have emphasized how women and men differ in terms of mental health and mental disabilities at work. According to international reports women have more mood-related disorders and they suffer more from mental-health-related work disabilities. In line with these findings, the number of sickness absence episodes due to mental disorders has been about double among working-age women compared to working-age men in Finland. A considerable gender difference is typically commented upon in statistical analyses and gender differences in the prevalence of symptoms and use of services is a standard in population-based reports. Given this context, it is surprising that underlying dynamics leading to such differences have been seldom addressed in occupational health research and contextualized from the analytical frameworks of gendered work and mental health (Annandale and Clark, 2008; Rikala, 2013; Pattyn, 2014).

Normalized gender perceptions of mental health research view men and women as natural and unequivocal categories. Women are usually portrayed as the 'sicker' sex, leading to greater use of mental health services (Courtenay, 2000; Addis and Mahalik, 2003). However, according to classical work by gender sociologists Candace West and Don Zimmerman (1987), gender should not be viewed as a naturalized category or even a social role, but rather as an accomplishment, the product of daily social practices and behaviours which manifest the subject's gender related identity and norms. Gender is performed, something which is 'done' in a continuing and context-related way. 'Doing gender' is established by means of interaction and is displayed through it, and while appearing as 'natural' it is something which is created by an organized social practice and official and non-official interactions.

Traditional research on emotion and gender differences between men and women has pointed out that women and men may hold different standards of 'appropriate' expressivity within the same interactional contexts (Chaplin, 2015). Stephanie Shields (2002: 21) uses a concept of gender-coded behaviour, which refers to a behaviour or experience that is expected to be more typical, natural and appropriate for one sex than the other. Doing gender in everyday life is closely connected to the perceptions, ideals and attitudes related to emotions and it is also applied as a way of understanding ourselves as gendered individuals (Shields, 2002: 55). Thus, doing gender through 'doing emotion' encompasses not only emotional display but also emotion values (for example, men express fewer emotions than women) and beliefs dealing with emotional experience (for example, low mood needs therapeutic support).

These theoretical frameworks suggest that managing mental health and emotions is intertwined with gendered social characters, as the 'silent man' reflected in the previous section. Because the core trajectories of mental vulnerability related to work ability seem to have a strong gender-related basis it is relevant to ask how mental health is reflected in gendered cultural standards and identities (Bohan, 1993; Connell, 1995; Courtenay, 2000) and whether distinctive manifestations of mental vulnerability are influenced by notions of gendered social and material conditions and doing gender (for example, Annandale et al, 2007).

Previous research in health sociology suggests that norms of masculinity and femininity determine how people respond to health problems in general. Robin Saltonstall (1993) has even proposed that the use of health services is a way to implement gender. Masculinity, femininity and, nowadays, increasingly also other diverse gender categories, affect health behaviour and, for example, the threshold to seek help when the mind is in distress (Annandale et al, 2007; Fleming and Agnew-Brune, 2015). Due to their strong interactional, narrated and subjective character (for example, Valkonen and Hänninen, 2013), it is plausible that mental vulnerabilities are especially interlinked with gendered subject positions and occupational practices taking place in gender-segregated contexts of work.

One way to analyse the role of gender in the context of mental health is to analyse it empirically from the perspective of ethnicity and cultural difference (for example, Kleinman et al, 1987). In one of our population studies, we found that most groups of working-age women with an immigrant background had considerably lower levels of psychotropic drug use and sickness absences due to mental health problems compared to women who had been born and raised in Finland (Bosqui et al, 2019, 2020). Perhaps the knowledge of mental health services was less developed in this group and language barriers could make the use of services more complex. However, the perspective of doing gender also leads us to ask if we are dealing with culture-specific gendered ways of coping with difficult emotions and psychological problems. For instance, among Somali, Kurdish, East-Asian and Eastern European women in Finland the psycho-emotional challenges do not seem to lead to mental health problems manifested in health registers to the same extent as in the general population. However, neither their occupational nor economic circumstances suggest a higher level of coping resources or less demanding everyday living conditions compared to their Finland-born counterparts, on the contrary (Olakivi et al, 2023).

Ellen Annandale (Annandale et al, 2007; Annandale and Clark, 2008), Stephanie Shields (2002) and Eduardo Bericat (2016) have analysed the social production of wellbeing and emotional reactions from the gender perspective. Based on these analyses, it could be suggested that current mental health practices such as use of selective serotonin reuptake inhibitors (SSRIs) and the treatment of social problems in psychotherapy are one way of constructing gender and especially femininity through emotional values and behaviours. Mental health discourses are used to build psyche-sensitive agency, which is especially related to the culture of self-care and the rise of middle-class emancipatory femininity in recent decades. In other words, psychological openness, emotional reflexivity, norms of sharing inner experiences and the active care of the mind can be viewed as idealized parts of gender-bound character idealizations.

Around 1960–2020, the value of emotional education (Ecclestone and Hayes, 2009) and mental capital (Cottingham, 2016) rose hand in hand with reformist movements, feminism and humanistic ideologies. These cultural shifts were accompanied by the humanization of work, radical psychiatry, ideals of minority and ethnic rights, and other approaches, stressing the subjective rights of individuals and promoting the importance of equality of wellbeing. In line with this, recent data-driven research has shown a considerable shift from the values of rationality to the values of emotionality over the past decades at least at the discursive level (Schmidt, 2021). These social changes have increased opportunities for self-expression and grievances among traditionally disadvantaged sections of the population in liberal Western countries. This observation suggests that gendered practices related to the management of the psyche and mental health could be viewed under the rise of an emotional imperative and emotion-driven solution-seeking. When viewed from the point of view of traditional gender categories, the strong gendered nature of mental health related to mood and emotions also seems to propose that cultural formalization of mental health is connected to behavioural repertoires that have been culturally more common among women. This suggests that it is reasonable to view psychological distress, work-related stress reactions and manifestations labelled as 'therapeutic' from the perspective of the historical continuum of gendered social characters and emotional practices.

Focus on sensitive care for oneself, therapeutic aid and more humane management can be viewed as a shift towards the recognition of a traditionally unofficial and feminine way of organizing emotional life. This can be seen as a cultural shift in societies long dominated by hegemonic masculinity (Connell, 1995; Schippers, 2007). An alternative, but equally relevant, interpretation is offered by sociologist Suvi Salmenniemi (2022: 186–187), who emphasizes that in Euro-American societies, a crucial element of self-sacrificing ethos for women has been the moral obligation to prioritize others' needs at the expense of one's own. She suggests that the current repertoire of mental health and therapeutic self-care may allow women to embrace vulnerability and legitimize care for and appreciation of the self. Although this may partly reflect a subordinate position, it is also likely to be linked to the wider democratization of emotional landscapes and social relations (Wouters, 2007).

As the psychological 'feel of the game' has become a more important dimension of the labour market, organizational contexts of doing gender have also been transformed. It can be argued that a need for psycho-emotional characteristics and qualities has formalized the importance of characteristics that are traditionally considered as feminine. This trend is clearly observable in the long-term transition of job advertisements (Kuokkanen et al, 2013; Varje et al, 2013a, 2013b): interactional and emotional capacities have gained importance and become sought-after aspects in the labour market. The change towards interaction-focused occupations (service, care, education) and job requirements has impacted the 'feminization' of organizational efficiency. In this setting, it not only became more expected and valued to create psychologically satisfying work cultures for all, but the same applied also to using emotions and psychological wellbeing as sources of profit-making (Hochschild, 2003 [1983]). As labour market demands tightened, medical-driven occupational health care increasingly began to treat the emotional problems of the female-dominated social and service sector through psychological tools and diagnostic language. Work stress, psychological distress, burnout and other aspects of emotional weariness rose as the importance of emotion-sensitive and human-orientated approaches were officially recognized both as an integral part of the moral value system and development of the workplace's capital.

Although social theoretical analyses of the gendered social order of emotions and health provide important analytical tools for the study of mental health in work, these analyses often miss the real-life conditions and subcultures of work. Gender may be marked by any of the other major categories of social identity such as age, occupation, ethnicity and region. According to Hochschild (1979, 2003 [1983]), there are culturally defined conventions for assessing the fit between emotion and the situation, and we make efforts to conform to these 'feeling rules'. If we understand mental health as a part of emotional behaviour of historical subjects, this also leads to the idea that mental health may be part of a collective system of emotional management in the gender-segregated labour market. According to Hochschild (2003 [1983]) and Shields (2002), we engage occupation-specific behavioural codes and feeling rules that are often viewed as an appropriate part of gendered occupational identity and social position.

But how are differences observed by employees themselves in the work community? This quote from one of our studies describes a typical argument employed by municipal workers in Finland:

Interviewer: Why do these problems present especially in female-dominated workplaces?

Respondent: Women can't let things go. If something happens in the work community, it gets talked, talked and talked about. And it's not just talking nicely, but talking behind someone's back, maybe even bad-mouthing in some work communities. And the things that happen, they go on and are argued about for so long that finally no one remembers the original reason why they started to squabble. (Early childhood education teacher, female)

The cultural characteristics related to feminine work communities are evidently present in our interview materials. Many commented that "there is a weird sort of dwelling and milling around … a certain kind of lamenting". It is possible to interpret these as stereotypical descriptions of female-dominated work communities, but the descriptions can also reflect something else. For example, it is possible that this type of gender-related differences in managing emotions reflect the way a female-dominated professional group reacts to problems at work as a collective from their gendered 'psychic landscape'

(Reay, 2005). All in all, this example illustrates how mental work ability-related habits, interpretations and attributions often have a strong communal dimension embedded in gender (Boysen et al, 2014; Milner et al, 2018).

At the same time, it is reasonable to take the view that lower social and organizational status can also produce gendered behavioural strategies that reflect disadvantaged position and perceived limited opportunities to influence at work. It is possible, therefore, that the rhetoric of women's communities reflects an attempt to take control of problems that are difficult in nature and beyond one's control.

'Yes, of course, there are privilege issues anyway, that it is still not quite the same to be a woman as a man in society. If you work in a position where you are not such a high-level expert, then it is more difficult to say about grievances, and there may also be a risk that no one else will say about them either.' (Technical specialist, female)

The formation of vulnerability is linked to class- and gender-bound behavioural resources and models. Mental vulnerability has a strong connection with the social character that is typical in certain population groups (Allen, 2004). Therefore, it is related to the challenges of everyday activities and habitual ways to solve them. For instance, well-educated professional women in Finland use some forms of mental health services, such as psychotherapy, relatively more compared to blue-collar women (Selinheimo et al, 2023), not to mention men, but this does not mean that they necessarily have more symptoms of poor mental health. In addition to differences in cultural and economic resources, it may also be the case that they feel special pressure to be mentally fit both at work and at home and seek professional help to support their coping. This example describes the multifaceted nature of vulnerability and socio-cultural differences in its manifestations.

Gender-differentiated occupational structures and available coping options give a macro-level context to the social characters associated with the mental vulnerability Year after year, they are visible, for example, as population group-specific mental health differences in health registers (Moriarty et al, 2009; Halonen et al, 2018a, 2018b). At the same time, region and other socio-spatial features contribute to the essence of distress and lead to distinctive social behaviours in relation to mental vulnerability (Veenstra, 2007). Overall, both socio-cultural and status-related characteristics influence the manifestation and development of mental health patterns in the population (Hakulinen et al, 2023).

It should be noted, however, that men in the same occupations seek professional help for psychological difficulties clearly less than their female colleagues (Kokkinen et al, 2023), whereas the use of alcohol and drugs continues to take a much more central position among working-age men in their repertoire of actions. Indeed, many observations suggest that observed gender differences are likely to be related to both socio-emotional strategies of acting in line with one's gender as well as resources of acting related to gender. In this way, 'doing difficult emotions' leads to the observed gender divide in the established indicators of mental health.

But how do the representatives of gendered occupations themselves view gender and the occupational culture in the formation of emotional coping strategies and mental vulnerabilities? Social work provides a good example as it has historically been considered women's work and the profession is dominated by women (Satka, 1995). In our archival study (Turtiainen et al, 2022), social workers gave ambivalent accounts regarding their work and its gendered nature. Some felt that social work itself was a gender-specific profession. They pondered whether female gender entailed inherent qualities for social work and its psychosocial requirements and its psycho-emotional job requirements. For example, they wondered if women had natural traits which augment their sense of 'compassion, closeness and the responsibility for their comrades' (Turtiainen et al, 2022). Others consider the impact of gender on how social workers struggle to cope with emotional problems. In this way, social workers themselves often generated explanations that suggest a complex interrelatedness between gendered obstacles of work and the skill requirements of the female-dominated field. Gender was seen to be intertwined with both the caring qualities of work and the emotional health risks of work.

Social work exemplifies how occupational structure, gender and mental vulnerability are interlinked. At the very centre of the welfare state there are various occupations mostly employing women which have high levels of mental health problems. In these occupations, mental strain is typical, the salary level is moderate or low, efficiency requirements have increased and the possibility to influence the working times or contents of the work are limited. Homecare assistants, social workers, nurses and other interactive human-orientated jobs are typically characterized by these features. Employees in these occupations use considerably more psychotropic medication and have a higher rate of mental health–related sickness absences than employees in most other occupations (Buscariolli et al, 2018; Kokkinen et al, 2019). Interestingly, however, men working in these occupations had also much higher levels of psychotropic drug use and mental-health-related sickness absences than other men, even though their level of mental health problems was lower than among their female counterparts working in the same occupations. This result is easily explained by the vulnerability of those entering the care and social professions. However, it is possible that gendered occupational conditions and sub-cultural practices can lead to significant differences between different groups of men in different occupations.

The workload that erodes work ability is also gendered when women and men are unequally divided into different occupations and working conditions. Poor status and experiences of scarcity often described in female-dominated sectors.

'We have even actually been banned from above to tell families that we have too few adults. While you yourself think that "how about child safety, we cannot act in this way." But we are instructed to smile and be flexible. At the same time, families get the impression that we are capable and then we are actually exhausted.' (Early childhood education teacher, female, born in the 1990s)

Occupations such as childcare and social work exemplify how emotionally demanding work, the structural pressures of society and gendered behaviours may generate the problematizations of mental health at work. To summarize, the variety and frequency of problems related to mental health manifested among women are therefore likely to be linked to measurable gender inequalities (for example, emotionally burdensome work, the glass ceiling, work–family conflict, economic resources).

Gendered social structures of behaviour seem to also be linked to the ideals of self-development and the spread of self-directness labelled under the title of 'individualization'. For instance, according to the Finnish Working Conditions Survey, the expansion of the subjective significance of all key spheres of life (family, work, leisure time) was more pronounced among women compared to men, and upper-white-collar women in particular, in the 2000s and 2010s (Sutela et al, 2019). Especially educated women seek personally meaningful life contents in various arenas of life more than men. It can be justly assumed that if life becomes overly filled with competing aspirations, the scarcity of time-related resources can turn life into a set of minute-to-minute schedules and an increasing acknowledgement of unreachable objectives. This may lead to 'weariness of the self' (Ehrenberg, 2010), and feelings of exhaustion and cynicism.

An alternative way is to look at what has stifled the emergence of mental health issues in male-dominated cultures. Historically oriented studies give hints about it. They have indicated, for example, how working-class male identity, daily habits and social roles have been limited the occupational health to the area of somatics (Turtiainen and Väänänen, 2012). Traditionally, male workers have respected the skills, strength and autonomy of their trade, but at the same time, the work and the habits and norms of the masculine industrial culture have been often harmful to their health. Hence, although the masculine ethos has helped men to overcome daily burdens and to find collective strength when needed, the behaviour has also been connected to risk-taking, and even with premature death (Dolan, 2011; Turtiainen and

Väänänen, 2012). In this context of strong masculinity, mental health has been silenced and its role in emotional coping has been narrow.

An interesting observation can be made when comparing different mental health indicators. Unlike other general mental health indicators such as anxiety, depression and use of psychotropic medication, women and men report symptoms of job burnout at a similar level (Purvanova and Muros, 2010). This may be related to a work-oriented social figure associated with masculinity, for whom exhaustion at work may be less stigmatizing than depression or other categories of psychiatry. Studies also indicate that men's mental vulnerability is linked to their labour market status, culture and social space. Bourdieu-inspired analyses, among others, show how the loss of important socio-material field, like in the case of long-term unemployment, men are easily deprived from valued masculine resources and their masculine identity is challenged (Robinson and Robertson, 2014). However, changes in masculine health behaviour are also noticeable as the latest health service statistics show how the youngest generations of men are more actively seeking professional psychological help (Social Security Institution of Finland, 2022b). Some recent observations from different industries also suggest that the concern about mental vulnerability has spread to industries considered masculine, such as construction. These observations describe the role of traditional work-related masculinity behind vulnerability, but on the other hand, they also indicate that masculinity could be at a turning point.

The analytical prism matters when examining gender and vulnerability. If we apply a work sociological stand and focus on municipal healthcare workers, childcare workers or social workers, we detect gendered occupational circumstances and demands as well as inferior power in society, which can be seen as fuelling mechanisms towards poor mental health. In contrast, if we apply the perspective of constructivist social sciences, and focus on upper educational classes, we end up with emotional displays, discourses, repertoires and narratives generating therapeutic dominance and the medicalization of everyday emotional life. However, from the perspective of mental vulnerability in daily life, the processes and mechanisms recognized by these scientific paradigms often overlap and co-occur. These observations propose that we need to analyse the occupation/gender-related ways of 'doing mental health and disability', applying theoretical perspectives that are relevant for their contexts. Gendered positions in the labour market and the area of wellbeing are likely to influence the way we identify mental vulnerabilities, name them, share them, intend to solve them and place them in the medical and non-medical settings.

Applying the perspective of social character and 'doing gender', it is reasonable to ask how the lives of working-age men and women are currently constructed so that it enables and/or requires women to act as vulnerable subjects with more psycho-emotional problems than men? To what extent does 'doing mental vulnerability' equate with doing gender? By generating these types of questions, we may also reach a somewhat novel framework for understanding the mental health crisis of our historical period. This suggests a research approach that intends to analyse how particular socio-cultural and economic frameworks of action generate vulnerable subjectivities and what is the role of gender in producing this. At the same time, it is worth noting how masculinity or femininity themselves are in transition and subject to a new kind of negotiation (Butler, 2006 [1990]). The change in gender will be closely related to what kind of position mental health will take in society and what role it will have in future work and work ability.

9

Mental vulnerability as a social practice

In this book, I have structured various professional and cultural paths that have led to the growth of a phenomenon I call mental vulnerability, especially in the labour market context. But how to describe the formation of vulnerability on a more general level? In this chapter, I will first describe how an approach that works at the individual level can produce increasing forms of vulnerability at the social level. Specifically, I analyse the individual/society contrast of vulnerability by considering the paradigm of strengthening individuals' mental-health-related and emotional awareness. Finally, I consider how the sources of mental vulnerability may relate to a very different type of experience of lack by distinguishing between two different types of scarcity characterizing current vulnerabilities.

Developing awareness – advancing vulnerability?

In the 2020s, psychotherapy and consciously taking care of one's mental wellbeing is much more usual than before. One could think that the development would lead to better mental health, but in most Western countries working-aged people report more mental health challenges than before. One way to approach this paradox is to analyse mental health from the point of view of social sharing and spreading of vulnerability at the cultural level. For example, current approaches emphasizing emotional literacy and mental health literacy reflect the increasingly common ethical guidelines available to employees, which emphasize an active relationship with one's own emotions and mental health. In this chapter, I describe how these approaches aimed at developing individual psycho-emotional consciousness reflect a new understanding of mental vulnerability and the social production of vulnerabilities in an individual-centred society.

In organizational studies David Hillson and Ruth Webster-Murray (2005, 2006) propose that the increasing importance of risks and emotional coping mechanisms, 'emotional literacy' using their terms, is intimately related to key aspects of workplaces and individuals. In their approach, they suggest that emotional literacy plays a growing role in the functioning of late modern organizations and the success of individual employees (Hillson and Murray-Webster, 2005). The approach consists of four components:

1. recognizing emotions, which includes, among other things, self-awareness, the ability to empathize and a trusting relationship with the work community;
2. understanding emotions, which includes, among other things, the ability to adapt one's own actions and trust in one's own actions and abilities;
3. expressing emotions appropriately, which includes, for example, goal-oriented emotional expression, emotional authenticity and openness, and the ability to give constructive criticism; and
4. managing emotions, which includes, for example, stress tolerance, controlling one's own impulses and taking care of one's own wellbeing.

These types of approaches propose that our current work culture requires the ability to detect various risks that surround us and may damage our functionality, both organizationally and personally. Furthermore, they propose that our emotional literacy skills essentially influence our capacity to view and estimate risks and uncertainties adequately and behave proactively. Finally, they offer us an intellectual framework which states that we need to develop our emotional literacy not only because we are supposed to understand and express emotions properly in current work but to manage our socio-emotional climate in the most optimal manner.

Based on our research with historical materials (Varje et al, 2013a; Väänänen and Turtiainen, 2014) and various studies on the sociology of risk (Van Loon, 2008; Wilkinson, 2009), the emotional literacy approach exemplifies a less acknowledged paradigm change of the 1990s and early 2000s in the popular understanding of work and workership. Namely, it reflects an 'ideal of proactive emotional management' based on a risk-focused future-orientated social character. This paradigm emphasizes how both the role of internal reflexivity and emotional capability are crucial building blocks of emotionally rational work behaviour that can and should use emotions as integral parts of one's personal development and organizational success (see also Bolton, 2005). Within these discourses, emotional skills, psychological interpretations and self-reflexivity are applauded

Not only has research on work and organizational educators promoted psycho-emotional literacy approaches. Already in the 1990s, Australian psychologist Anthony Jorm et al (1997) introduced the term 'mental health literacy' and defined it as 'knowledge and beliefs about mental disorders which aid their recognition, management or prevention'. Mental health literacy consists of several components, including:

• the ability to recognize specific disorders or different types of psychological distress;
• knowledge and beliefs about risk factors and causes;
• knowledge and beliefs about self-help interventions;

- knowledge and beliefs about professional help available;
- attitudes which facilitate recognition and appropriate help-seeking; and
- knowledge of how to seek mental health information.

To sum up, idealized skills of mental health boosting and buffering include acknowledgement, identification, activity and self-help skills. For example, the timely use of mental health services are encouraged. The active use of psychological treatments such as psychological counselling (McKeon and Carrick, 1991; Jorm et al, 2000, 2006) and psychotherapy (Hillert et al, 1999) are indicators of having a good mental health literacy. The perspective suggests that by raising general knowledge on psychological, medical and healthy lifestyle related issues, it is possible to best treat mental malaise (Jorm et al, 1997). In this way, the conceptual history of mental health literacy is connected to the wider concept of health literacy, which aims to increase individual knowledge of physical health, illnesses and treatments. From the perspective of critical history of sciences, it belongs to the same group of concepts as emotional intelligence, resiliency, self-efficacy and other similar concepts. All these concepts aim to strengthen societal and/or organizational vitality by rationally impacting individuals' emotional capabilities and psychological resources.

At this point in the history of work-related behaviour and health, the literacy frameworks aim to improve people's capacity via providing more knowledge and tools that inhibit irrational and unhealthy behaviours (for example, turning inwards, self-harm, adopting a negative self-image). As such, these frameworks targeted at the improvement of emotional and mental skills are based on the humanist ideal that people ought to be guided towards a better life by providing new understanding and tactical information on emotions, mental illnesses and their appropriate management. But how are these cultural and organizational trends related to mental vulnerability?

I consider these approaches focused on the development of psychological self-navigation and training self-management to be important for the analysis of mental vulnerability. For instance, according to the paradigm, the social character should be emancipatory, capable of making decisions and setting meaningful goals, future-oriented, and able to empower oneself by using psychological and medical information and services. In other words, these knowledge-enhancing paradigms promote a normative ideal of a proactive rational subject who is capable of making psychologically healthy and proactive decisions and view their situation from the perspective of mental wellbeing and mental health. In this way, these approaches promote an ideal that each one of us ought to be better copers and capable of using various types of psycho-emotional frameworks. At the societal level, the development of such an individual-oriented citizen, who actively treats himself with psychological tools, is likely to lead to mental health issues becoming more and more prominent both at work and in other areas of life. Through this, these models of thinking may have significant unintended societal influences that may be more significant than the original aims of these projects and their behavioural ideals if they become commonly used.

The development of managing and guiding emotions and the psyche can be seen as an extension of the 'health gaze' into the social sphere of social behaviour and individual responsibility. If a Foucauldian analysis is followed, as a form of mental health gaze, awareness approaches redefine the cultural mindset by drawing a line between healthy behaviour and risky behaviour. These approaches craft social existence into risk factors that must be confronted with appropriate organizational and health behaviours and politics (see also Armstrong, 1995).

Nikolas Rose (2007: 465–466) has interestingly defined that many psychiatric disorders have become 'disorders without borders', because psychological knowledge can be grown indefinitely in society. Similarly, the Finnish sociologist Ilpo Helén (2007b) has proposed that the broadening of the epidemiological approach and mental health paradigm has meant a change towards mental health risks and risk factors which should be somehow managed and prevented. Within this framework, the focus has shifted to individual life management skills. Also in our own studies, the strengthening of the perspective of the awakened individual has come to the fore, for example, in the Finnish insurance industry, as it has turned towards emphasizing individual responsibility and self-control of stress since the 1990s. The spreading of mental health awareness, which is limitless in nature, also means new ethical guidelines for how people are thought to be able to achieve a good life (Rose, 1996; Miller and Rose, 2008; Kinnunen, 2020a). In an individual-oriented society and science, using various emotional and self-management skills is increasingly recognized as a natural part of correct and smart behaviour. It is obvious that therapy consulting companies, psychological coaching services, mental health organizations and the psychopharmacological industry have their own goals and an important role in this development.

Psycho-emotional toolkits and awareness skills are solutions designed and sold to a society of autonomous individuals without a stable social compass. Identity-driven self-management calls for proactive psychological interventions and self-understanding. The mental load rising from the orchestration of the psyche and norms of active emotional work encourages a growing number of employees into psychological approaches, therapeutic solutions and medical advice-seeking. Hence, the transition towards mental vulnerability has not only occurred due to the change of work: the potentially vulnerable mind needs much stronger attention than before due to the cultural transitions of the social character.

The transition towards the recognition and management of subjectivities among individuals also signifies the entrance of a new cultural ethos that has situated and invested much higher value in personal experiences, narratives and individual interpretations. Emotional wellbeing, intrinsic motivation, experiences of bullying, social climate and other themes related to subjective experiences and emotions became far more significant around 1980–2020 than in the earlier period of work culture. This was one of the central forces that began to produce new speech, classification and social action that I have described in this book as mental vulnerability.

The turn towards mental vulnerability took place along with new knowledge paradigms, emotional management norms and a generational transition. The public and occupational health culture related to a framework of mental health and various treatments supporting it gradually changed and started to emphasize actively working with mental health (Dew et al, 1991; Jorm, 2000). In the context of work, more mental health professionals were required to treat work ability problems, and new programmes related to mental health promotion were launched. Currently, the new kind of limitlessness of mental health is reflected in the activities of several working-age population groups through, for example, mental health education and the teaching of emotional skills (Ecclestone and Hayes, 2009). Some social critics have taken the nihilistic view that in a psychological society based on psychoeducation, the greatest use of power is often presented as a form of liberation and empowerment (Smith, 1997; Tunestad, 2014).

Philosopher Timothy Morton (2016) speaks about 'ecognosis', the strange process of knowledge production in current societies, a knowing that knows itself (see also Braidotti, 2019: 83). Even though Morton focuses on environmental knowing in his analysis, I see a link with mental vulnerability. In the late modern society of fast communication, the vulnerability of the subject and the knowledge about it are in a dialectical relationship. The ecology of mental health is a dynamic system where knowledge takes place in various social networks and belief systems in which subjective self-awareness and collective knowledge on potential vulnerability feed each other. Self-awareness arises from social knowledge. Risk discourses spread rapidly and leave us with awareness of our vulnerability. This presents us with a paradox situation: whereas the rationale underlying preventive medicine and various strands of applied psychology is the protection against our vulnerability as humans, the development of consciousness, emphasis on emotional experience and adaptation related to continuous changes also create constant reminders of human vulnerability (see also Skolbekken, 2008: 19). Over the past two decades, the strong evolvement of mental health forums has contributed to the amplification of looping effects (social media, digital channels, services), potentially impacting social vulnerability.

Cultural products provide one way to identify the dynamics of these literacies as part of cultural understanding. In the sarcastic documentary *The Happy Worker* by John Webster (2022), today's office workers with their market-driven mental suffering are described from the perspective of job burnout. Pretence, overwhelming tasks and collective chimera are among the main topics of this documentary. The film addresses the typical drawbacks of white-collar jobs and organizations in the early 2020s globally affecting hundreds of millions of employees. The protagonists of the film participate in peer group sessions for burnout survivors and one of the leading work psychologists, Christina Maslach, presents her views and interpretations. Although the macro framework of grievances is recognized, the phenomenon is defined through the language of burnout and mental health while psychology and micro-group-level interventions are provided as solutions to the audience. Consequently, these types of cultural products, even critical ones, can provide support to knowledge-seeking based on individual risk management and proactivity. At the same time, they are likely to stimulate conceptualizations and attributions stressing the burdening experiences of the individuals and increase demands for new mental health services supporting the individuals (see also Brinkmann, 2016).

Philosophers of science such as Ian Hacking (1999) have observed looping effects in the construction of knowledge in the social and behavioural sciences. In the context of societal change, burnout, depression and work stress constitute 'a moving target' (Hacking, 1999: 144), whose definitions and criteria change as transitions in the surrounding society and work are reflected on them (Giddens, 1984). In effect, there is constant interactive feedback between the science of work-related health and its object so much that the categories of science, such as psychiatric categories, continue to change (Danziger, 1997: 193). From the point of view of social behaviour and perceived challenges of work, research on mental health and work is therefore not 'independent' since people and cultural products (for example, documentaries on work) interpret and adopt psychological and psychiatric concepts and classifications of the current era. On the other hand, categories and concepts related to work ability and mental health have an interactive relationship with our mental lives, shaping and colouring as well as explaining them (see Dixon, 2012: 338; Newton, 2022).

The looping processes are manifested in workplaces (anticipation of vulnerability), educational institutions (development of mental health awareness) and identity-forming (identification of one's vulnerability). The subject may both benefit from these conceptualizations in their everyday life or work but simultaneously recognize new vulnerabilities that remained disregarded and silenced in the earlier historical periods. Consequently, looping effects underlie the self-developmental and self-caring aspect of current mental health and emotional management. Discursive plurality focusing on mental vulnerability have become elemental parts of this cultural landscape in which vulnerabilities are identified, discussed and treated.

The dynamic between the collective awareness of the importance of mental health and the new reflexive social character have generated the troublesome mental health in late modernity. The continuous impacts of the looping effects are something that the late modern 'sovereign self' who is above all on 'its *own* ground' has to deal with (Dunne, 1995: 137). The continuous publicity of a self-focused psycho-emotional character is manifested in psychology-orientated autobiographies and narratives of mental health recovery. One decisive moment towards working and pondering on the psyche in the Finnish context took place in the late 1990s when a famous theatre director and scriptwriter, Neil Hardwick, publicly described his depression in the media and when the spouse of ex-president Tellervo Koivisto openly explained her episodes of depression on television. During the same period a national survey showed how a considerable part of the working-age population suffered from severe job burnout. In the early 2000s, the debate about depression spread and national mental health interventions were launched.

The mental health testimonies by famous people were mostly seen positively and were warmly welcomed in a country that had grown into a national self-understanding of silence and introversion. Previously unspoken matters were transformed into words and various expressions of mental suffering became more socially acceptable. However, simultaneously, the need for self-management and redirection of unpleasant affective states of the autonomous and self-reflective individuals increased, and new practices of care were sought. From the point of view of the historical turning point of the psyche, new treatment practices (for example, brief therapy) and the strong increase in the use of antidepressants between the 1990s and 2020s is a natural part of the transition. They reflect the development of a social character that is more autonomous and self-aware, and the shift of the focus of behaviour to the area of mood control and self-direction. From this perspective, the triumph of positive paradigms (for example, engagement, flow, efficacy) has partly the same source as the mental health crisis among the working-aged. It is the result of an increase in the value of psychological experience and the development of emotion-oriented individuality.

But how significant is this paradigm of psychological knowledge in everyday interactions? Is it mainly an ideal of individualistic sciences? One way to approach the situation is offered by Australian scholar of psychology, Nick Haslam (2005), according to whose results 'psychologizing mental health problems' is currently one of the central ways to understand mental health. Psychologization signifies that psychological concepts and approaches are commonly applied in the everyday explanations and definitions of mental health at least in many Western societies (Pescosolido et al, 1998; see also

Rose, 2007). According to our results, various sources describing good workership (Varje et al, 2013a) and occupational health (Väänänen et al, 2014; Varje and Väänänen, 2016) have indeed shifted towards psychological concepts and explanation models since the 1960s. It could be summarized that if the psychotechnics of work in the early 20th century aimed at maximizing the worker's output and shaping the soul into a non-political form, after the 1960s the psychological view on subjectivity was able to sneak in, in the form of an emancipated employee with a psychologically attuned way of understanding themselves and their wellbeing.

Many historical materials of work describe how the professionals of the past era were no longer suited to the new era. The loss of worker value brought about by the labour market and technological change was increasingly addressed by turning to the individual's emotions and strengthening psychological capacity. A work identity that had lost its value led to mental-health-related disability through difficult emotional processes. For instance, the essential character forms of masculine industrial workers of the post-war era experienced considerable crisis in the late 20th century when automatization and globalization began to undermine traditional work contents and ways of working. Since the 1990s in particular, the structural change manifested itself as pressure in healthcare and a new kind of demand to expand mental health. The conflictual historicity of social being (subjectivity) and becoming (ideals concerning emotional subjectivity) has culturally framed the question of the mental vulnerability.

The analyses of late modernity often place particular emphasis on the emergence of a reflexive social character (for example, Giddens, 1991; Archer, 2012), whose behaviour and preferences are not determined by traditions and small-scale communities. This figure is often portrayed in the sociology of work as a person generated by a labour market that lives in constant change and is characterized by reorientation and flexibility. For instance, when describing late modern project work carried out by millions of employees, Luc Boltanski and Eve Chiapello (2007) analysed the project-based way of self-organizing in which life is conceived as a succession of projects. Within this 'polis', a person's value is measured by the activity they perform. According to this interpretation, passivity and routines are an enemy of the entrepreneurial self, moving from one project to another. Although the analysis of the project-based polis may overstate the role of work processes when it comes to mental vulnerability, it does capture the economic and organizational background underlying individual-oriented literacy instructions.

Psychological literacy skills and self-directed control of emotional activity arise from a genuine need. Organizations and employees have come under pressure to find means to cope with increasing unpredictability and navigating in life. The ability to adapt and the potential to change are needed. Critical scholars argue that we are dealing with the 'politics of stretching' (Honkasalo, 2018). The demands of the cognitive economy require organizational and psychological flexibility. However, not all people (or all of the time) are able to adapt to these demands and expectations. The demands of the flexible economy create a need for a politics of vulnerability, because the stretching of limits is likely to create unwanted side-effects in the form of distress, irresolution and agony. At this point, emotional literacy skills, self-compassion, controlling the mind and other similar tools have stepped in as ways to ease the burden on the psyche.

In the face of the amazing rise of mental health problems, mainly researchers of therapization (Furedi, 2004; Ecclestone and Hayes, 2009), psychiatrization (for example, Beeker et al, 2021) and psychologization (for example, Madsen, 2018) have gained popularity. I think that these analyses are often insightful in the field dominated by individual explanations, but they have made me ask: How about work-related health and disability over the past 50 years? How about different groups of workers and professionals, problems described by them, their circumstances, and their views? In the research materials, actors representing different occupations seem to respond to the demands of their time in a manner relevant to themselves and their community. The changes we have found have often been related to the evolution of the occupation, and psychological information has been adopted quite differently in different parts of the labour market. Therefore, the range of changes also urges us to critically examine cultural sociological analyses of the link between a psychological worldview and mental vulnerability (Elias, 1991, 1994).

Based on the analyses, it could be concluded that psychology and psychological understanding have provided material (for example, concepts, measures, intervention tools) for the identification and management of vulnerability. At the same time, individualistic awareness-promoting approaches have also begun to frame the phenomenon with psychological concepts. However, it is important to note that the development has been heterogeneous and psychological knowledge has been adopted at quite different levels in different locations of the labour market. The general hypothesis of psychologization does not hold for some employment sectors (Turtiainen and Väänänen, 2012; Lehmuskoski et al, 2022), and the profiles of mental health behaviour imply differences in terms of use of psychological solutions (Halonen et al, 2018a; Eggenberger et al, 2021). Our study of young working adults in the 2020s also shows how ways to manage psycho-emotional stress vary even within the generation commonly classified as a problematic group (Lehmuskoski et al, 2022).

Finally, it is important to note that the dominant conception of mental health and its management influences the politics of mental vulnerability. A good example of this is a research project we carried out for the Finnish Prime Minister's Office (Ervasti et al, 2022). We conducted an extensive scientific review that showed how studies on mental-health-related support measures aimed at strengthening work ability are almost exclusively performed at the individual level. A vast majority of the studies focused on the impact of methods such as stress management, lifestyle interventions and recovery suggestions. Across the studies, the measures of mental health were found to be individual based, indicated by depressive symptoms, psychiatric sick leaves and psychotropic medication use which were seen as markers of psychological disability or mental health challenges. Similar examples from international research show how both practical activities in the field of work ability and mental health as well as the mainstream mental health research carried out guide the topic of mental vulnerability into a personal matter and into the framework of individual-level solutions. At the same time, the role of labour market transitions and cultural change becomes blurred. Instead of asking questions about the sources of increased mental vulnerability, they start measuring the mental health of individuals and evaluate the possibilities of changing it in the light of research data. It is a serious structural challenge both in terms of science and politics.

The dual engines of mental vulnerability

Based on many materials, the source of mental vulnerability may be in both traditional inequality and struggling with the orientation of one's own psychoemotional management. Next, I will describe two extremes in a late modern society, where mental vulnerability arises for various reasons. These extremes seek to clarify how the sources of vulnerability fundamentally differ, varying according to populations and circumstances. Since both extremes are about opportunities for action that are perceived to be weak for various reasons, and often even outright deprivation of meaningful future prospects, I have named the extremes Scarcity 1 and Scarcity 2. The area of Scarcity 1 includes traditional disadvantage, material deprivation and the need for perseverance produced by a weak social position. Its counterpart is Scarcity 2, which in turn is characterized by challenging thoughts and feelings arising from the difficulty of realizing subjective goals and objectives. The experience easily gives rise to negative feelings and hopes for something better.

In late modern society, Scarcity Type 1 is often associated with increasing efficiency, increasingly redundant skills and the burden of mismatch between the demands of work and the available skill resources of the population. It points to people who have difficulties in meeting the demands and requirement of work and production. These people are often located on the lower ladder of income and their work is often carefully monitored and pre-organized. Many of them float between work and non-work and/or work when there happens to be an available job. This kind of scarcity is often present in platform work, zero-hour contracts, various forms of involuntary part-time employment and a wide range of low-wage work characterized by low resources and challenging work conditions. In the most severe situations are often those populations who intend to survive in the informal economy applying strategies of improvisational survivalism in their daily life (Eriksen, 2016). In most Western societies welfare institutions are needed to support these 'populations at risk' or 'vulnerable populations'. Nevertheless, several epidemiological studies show how material poverty, low social and occupational status and poor integration in work play a decisive role in the formation of mental health challenges (Lahelma et al, 2006; Muntaner and Chung, 2007; Eaton et al, 2010).

However, extensive social scientific research also points out how mental vulnerabilities in the workforce do not only emerge from agony, frustration and stress caused by material reality and over-taxing work conditions. Vulnerability also has a socio-behavioural background. According to observations made by Ehrenberg in France, Côté in North America, Brinkmann in Denmark, Madsen in Norway, Illouz in Israel, MacLaughlin in England, our research group in Finland and many other researchers in other countries, the analysis of late modern subjectivity needs to be included in the social diagnosis of the mental health crisis. From the perspective of the social history of individualization in Western countries, these tendencies of vulnerability can be seen as part of a long continuum of conflicts arising from the development of modern identity and the birth of the late modern self (for example, Baumeister, 1986; Giddens, 1991), including the transition from traditional external control to internal control and self-management. In this historical macro-context, the search for the contents of life and work tasks that correspond to our inner self has been an increasingly central part of the shared reality in which we have lived since the late 1900s. The scarcity associated with the inaccessibility of self-desires that are considered personal and the need for psychological inner work belongs to the other extreme of the scarcity polarity, the area of Scarcity Type 2.

The nature of Scarcity Type 2 easily leads to intrapsychic expeditions and trying to shape one's life individually in a direction that feels right. In this book, I have associated this with three socio-cultural trends. First, psychological humanism and its popularizations have paved a way for self-focused values and needs for self-development. Second, the democratization of social relationships and the dissolution of social hierarchies (pupils versus teachers, patients versus doctors, and so on) has made it possible for different population groups and new generations to have more autonomous subjectivities who prefer self-determination and self-aware life management. Third, the individualization related to the search for subjectively meaningful work in the macro context of limited opportunities has emphasized the individual's mentally burdening experiences while the use of psychological filters has increase the recognition of psycho-emotional burdens. In this way, it seems even natural that the challenges arising from individuality are often labelled as 'identity work', 'lack of motivation', 'dissatisfaction with work' or 'existential life crises'. Consequently, they are also typical cultural channels for drifting towards looking for solutions in mental health talk and mental health systems.

As in the case of Scarcity Type 1, there seems to be a desire for better future and lack of tools to achieve the goal. However, the fundamental nature of shortage is not material but psycho-emotional. The future seems to be drifting away or blurring as the individual tries to approach it. In the context of work, the contemporary gaze is increasingly turned to the match between one's work and psycho-emotional objectives. In this social context, there are populous groups of working-age people who try to avoid the trap of getting stuck in unpleasant and poorly rewarding personal and organizational situations. The risk of uncomfortable and psychologically exhausting subjectivity is also intended to be resolved in the context of mental health by using professional help.

In the context of work, Scarcity Type 2 often entails a conflict between standards of professionalism and the lack of adequate resources to reach these internalized aims in occupational life characterized by poor organizational resources and the mantra of making profit. Social anthropologist Thomas Hylland Eriksen (2016: 116) states that there seems to be a growing contradiction between universal human rights and the neoliberal creating of human value on an economic scale. There seems to also be a psychological contradiction between widely promoted ideals of identity-corresponding life goals repeated in adolescence (find your thing, listen to yourself) and the scarcity of resources and/or the economy's profit-seeking maximization of the profit made with human capacities. This leads to the subjective and endogenic nature of Scarcity Type 2 which is less observable in Scarcity Type 1. In other words, psychological misfit and value incongruence perceived at work (for example, Doblhofer et al, 2019) may be increasingly felt when valued social positions are unreachable and unsatisfactory options in the form of work task, career and future prospects are perceivable. In many of our qualitative studies of Finnish workers, this phenomenon related to psychological discomfort and the shattering of ideals has been clearly noticeable (Väänänen et al, 2020; Lehmuskoski et al, 2022; Turtiainen et al, 2022).

The macro-psychological historical perspective on the recent past also provides an opportunity to understand the intertwining between the two types of scarcity. Related to the historical construction of Scarcity Type 2, and partly also Scarcity Type 1, cultural theorist Lauren Berlant (2011) has analysed how Europe and the United States wore away the fantasies of upward mobility associated with the liberal state since the 1980s. According to her interpretation there has been a decline of various institutionalized ideologies such as social equality, welfare, hard work and career progress. Life is increasingly characterized by unachievable fantasies of the good life.

This has led to 'cruel optimism'. It manifests itself as a relational dynamic in which individuals created attachment towards desired object-ideas in their behaviour even when the conditions for flourishing and fulfilling such promises are unrealistic. A relation of cruel optimism exists when something you desire is unreachable or even an obstacle to your flourishing. It might be a fantasy of good life, a political project, a desired job, or a new habit that promises to induce in you an improved way of being. These types of optimistic relations become cruel when the object that draws your attachment impedes the aim that brought you to it initially. According to Berlant's analysis, committing to object-ideas that sustain the good life fantasy, no matter how cruel these attachments may be, might allow people to make it through day-to-day life even though the day-to-day has become challenging.

Cruel optimism offers an important psychocultural explanation for the surge of new vulnerabilities in the context of contemporary therapeutic encounters which often deal with the impossibility of fulfilling the hopes for self-realization and self-satisfying life objectives (Marques, 2018). Therapeutic encounters thus receive inputs from the crisis of psychological humanism, but at the same time they are part of this crisis and its core. Portuguese social scientist Thiago Marques (2018) summarizes the importance of this analysis from the perspective of health research: 'Critical analyses of illness and health must account for the forms of suffering emerging not only in the context of poverty but also in contexts of precariousness, individualism, the dissolution of social support networks, and the erosion of welfare state protections.'

The dual nature of scarcity embodies the social relativity of mental vulnerability. Already in the 1960s, British sociologist Peter Townsend (Townsend, 1962: 210) argued that both poverty and subsistence can only be defined in relation to the material and emotional resources available at a particular time to the members either of a particular society or different societies. In his seminal study on poverty in the United Kingdom he noted:

> Individuals, families and groups in the population can be said to be in poverty when they lack the resources to obtain the types of diet, participate in the activities and have the living conditions and amenities which are customary, or are at least widely encouraged and approved, in the societies to which they belong. Their resources are so seriously below those commanded by the average individual or family that they are, in effect, excluded from ordinary living patterns, customs and activities. (Townsend, 1979: 31)

What is essential for the development of mental vulnerability in this definition is the historical and social contextual nature of scarcity. As cultural beings, people structure their own position and desires in relation to the community that is essential to them and its history. The relational nature of mental vulnerability signifies that different generations, genders, ethnic groups and socio-economic sub-sections of the population have different views and visions in relation to different categories of scarcity. These differences are also easily manifested in moral principles regarding the criteria for work disability and in terms of means for coping with social and emotional difficulties. They are also illustrated in the organizational practices, narrative accounts and cultural habits of handling psychological hardships. The increasing subjectivity of scarcity in the contemporary labour market also signifies that it is challenging to evaluate the severity of manifestations of mental vulnerability across populations, because the criteria vary and fluctuate.

As austerity measures have tightened and capitalism's desire for flexibility has increased, a growing number of people have found themselves between Scarcity Types 1 and 2. For instance, care and education work are characterized by strong social and emotional pressure but limited resources to change the situation. It can be justly argued that the cynicism felt by nurses is not necessarily related to burnout syndrome but lack of adequate resources of work, whereas the lowered threshold of irritability among teachers may not have to do with depressive symptomology but a pile of illegitimate work tasks (Rikala, 2014). Professional ideals and personal life-course objectives concerning work and its fundamental purpose is often contested by organizational reality. There is an abundance of identity projects in a context in which material wealth and professional resources no longer increase and subjective life goals taste of compromise. The conflict between personal objectives and exogenous resources chafes and the limited set of resources available to strive for psychological meaningful aims cause dissatisfaction. Workplaces do not work on the principle that the maximum number of people can realize their potential. The finite options push self-realization onto shaky ground. In the conflict between social character idealizations and lack of sufficient resources, mental health approaches are easily mobilized. Consequences are present in questionnaire responses and declining statistics regarding mental-health-related work ability.

In repository datasets of historical archives, people born in the late 1800s and early 1900s typically described not being able to go to school or enter the profession they wanted. This was often due to poverty, poor starting points, community peer pressure and a very limited range of occupations. Recently, the criteria at the base of scarceness experience have changed focus. Now, for many, a major criterion is no longer freeing oneself from the ropes of poverty but achieving cultural and self-related ideals. If we consider the whole population, vulnerability is not increased principally because of economic uncertainty or small controlling communities, but by the intersectional processes related to the transition of work, de-hierarchization of culture, and ever-escaping ideals of subjectivity. More and more people end up in a situation where help for the problems of the burdened psyche is sought from various social and knowledge-based expert forums.

Taking into account the transformation of work and subject, it is justified to propose that recently emerged interactional and/or information-focused work generates vulnerability under the conditions of late modernity, because these work characteristics resonate with the psyche committed to self-development. At the individual level, this can manifest itself in feelings of inadequacy, anxiety, frustration and desires for change. This dynamic is what Ehrenberg describes as the weariness of the self.

Interestingly, already more than 120 years ago sociologist Georg Simmel (1950 [1903]) described the newly emerged social character of modernity as follows: 'The carrier of man's values is no longer the "general human being" in every individual, but rather man's qualitative uniqueness and irreplaceability.' However, the analysis of the delayed modernization of Finland shows how modernization has not been a linear process and has progressed towards self-development among others at different speeds and times in different sectors of the society. Autonomous individuality with specific life goals and the quest for self-realization has been manifested more widely not only at work but also in various social forums and public discussions since the 1960s. For instance, women's magazines and media outlets were the promoters of the new modern figure (Nordberg, 2022). The features of modern subjectivity with psychological characteristics, ego-focused projects and individualist aspirations gradually spread to Finnish society as the society was urbanized, the welfare state developed, small-scale communities withered, consumer culture evolved, and work provided new opportunities. A new set of social codes, skills and processing channels for the self were called for in a new cultural environment.

For me, it was an arresting experience when I talked to my own aunt about everyday life and people in her childhood family some years ago. I tried to somehow get to grips with people's characters in my family in the 1940s. I received a surprising answer to my inquiries. She contested: "We didn't think about those things then!" The view of life dictated by material scarcity was at odds with an individual-oriented idea of man that evaluated the characteristics and psychological traits of individuals. Similar observations regarding intergenerational differences have also been made by researchers who have studied long-term social character transformations and historical changes in viewing life (Roos, 1987; Häkkinen and Salasuo, 2016). They pinpoint the significance of local history and shared social norms in people's possibilities of action and ways of understanding everyday life at different times.

This analysis points both to the social grievances and the transition of being a self. In the labour market, there is traditional scarcity and inequality, as well as a predicament related to individualization. The engines of vulnerability arising from various sources produce a fluctuation of the emotional compass at the individual level and a constant need to reflect on one's own direction. At this point in history, concepts and belief systems such as mental health are integrated into the behavioural repertoire. At the same time, the consequences of the change in work and culture are increasingly being solved in the management systems of psychological health and work ability. In this way, the rise of mental vulnerability at work is thus part of a long-term cultural and economic process, where the histories of work and cultural subjects intersect and produce change in employee ideals, standards of work ability and limits of health.

10

The temporal nature of mental health at work

By using various empirical materials and approaches from different disciplines, this book has sought to expand the understanding of how the working-age population has turned to mental health challenges. I have located various, often paradoxical, changes that have pushed the phenomenon of mental vulnerability to the fore. However, is it possible to say something general and sufficiently analytical about the change without diminishing the local character of mental vulnerabilities and the multiple processes fuelling it? Next, my aim is to compile a summary of key changes that have influenced the emergence and formation of vulnerability. After this, I consider the possibilities of integrating the social subject into the field of studies of the psyche and work, and describe how overlapping social transformations have produced a social setting and practice that I call wellness medicine. Finally, I examine mental health as a social ritual of our time.

The key elements of mental vulnerability

This section of the book places the key observations concerning work, work ability, emotional coping and mental health in the historical continuum (Alvesson, 2001; Amabile et al, 2005; Mookherjee, 2005; Ybema et al, 2009). Based on the materials and analyses presented in this book, I suggest that the current generations have moved to a new space of behaviour and experiences, in which mental vulnerability and subjective experiences have acquired a new status and social role. The first change is the transition to the era of wellbeing emphasizing broader non-material subjective health. The second one is the transformation of the work and labour market, demanding, utilizing and consuming psychological and emotional qualities. The third change is related to the fact that, with the breakdown and individualization of the social status-based lifeworld, managing the psyche has become a key challenge in late modern society. In conclusion, several parallel processes have moved us towards a new structural (for example, language, society's services) and experiential (for example, personal criteria, preferences, goals) reality in our work and understanding of the psyche, where managing vulnerability plays an essential part (cf Williams, 1980; Lee and Wrench, 1987). This framework is summarized in Figure 10.1.

Figure 10.1: The socio-historical framework of mental vulnerability

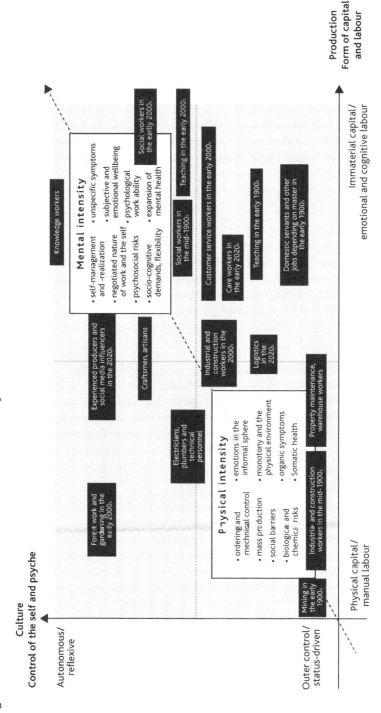

Figure 10.1 describes how the evolution of mental vulnerability can be understood by placing it in the arena between production and culture. This framework of mental vulnerability illustrates how we are moving away from physical work and material concerns and shifting towards mental work and emotional concerns characterized by socio-cognitive demands and psychological understanding. Instead of manual production, mechanical control, hierarchical power relations, somatic health problems and a narrow mental illness approach, work and social life are increasingly characterized by the democratization of social relationships, autonomous functioning and the liberalization of emotional challenges. As Figure 10.1 suggests, the change has not been linear. The employee's position in the labour market and other cultural and economic frameworks of behaviour have influenced how and to what extent the growth of mental intensity and its repositioning have begun to produce different manifestations of vulnerability. In Figure 10.1, I have used a few examples from different occupations and historical eras in order to describe the change.

The general progress of modernization has impacted how people view others and themselves. I have analysed this using the concept of social character. The modernization of social character models has impacted possibilities and standards that are viewed as relevant in the communities. The forms of social character are reflected, for instance, in the ideals of good workers, appropriate coping methods in difficult situations, and the role of subjective wellbeing among individuals. Dominating forms of social character illustrate the observed limits and possibilities of being and becoming a worker and/or subject in a given historical period. Social character formations also rule out alternatives of social action that are framed as impossible, undesirable or unrecognizable for economic or cultural reasons. For instance, during the processes of modernization, employees started to apply more science-driven concepts and narratives, value social behaviour based on norms of equality and negotiation, as well as understand psychological wellness as a crucial part of their social existence and as important criteria for a good working life.

Materials from a variety of employment sectors indicate that mental vulnerability has not developed in the same way everywhere. Examples drawn from teaching, insurance sales and social work demonstrate how the key resources valued in the production and work processes have changed and taken their own paths over the decades. New social settings with new skill requirements have evolved in various occupations and completely new frameworks of work have emerged. In 1970–2020 most sectors of employment also experienced layoffs and other reductions while intending to gear production towards improved efficiency, measuring profits quarterly and monitoring with more detail. Many previously valid skills were no longer needed, and the new wounds started to be treated in the area of occupational mental health.

As material welfare and occupational safety progressed, accident-inducing environments or lack of adequate housing were no longer the crucial sources of concern but the expending of numerous social and cognitive demands, growth of clientele, demands of making profit and constant changes at the workplace became typical work-related worries. At the same time, no longer were the monotony of industrial production or mechanical repetition of the same tasks the most common features of unpleasant work but challenges of abstract work, interpersonal demands and the problems with continuous self-management became new challenges.

The position of the psyche in work has changed: the emphasis on the connection between mental wellbeing and productivity has become more essential in growing numbers of workplaces as production has become interaction- and knowledge-based. The importance of mental and social capital is increasingly emphasized in job descriptions and organizational goals. Unlike traditional mental health, the new mental health is psychological potential and emotional reserve produced by sleep, exercise, relaxation, social relationships and other restorative and vitality promoting actions of the individual. In this psychological economy, psychological capacities and positive emotions are highlighted as a key component of success with slogans such as 'people make the organization' and 'human capital'.

Due to these transitions in the behavioural arenas of society and subjectivity itself, employees, workplaces, labour market organizations, patient organizations and politicians have awakened. The interaction between the demands of production and the sensitized psyche creates a need for protection and support mechanisms at the individual level. In individual-centred societies, people turn to medical and psychological solutions, because medical and psychological forums are considered to be legitimate solution platforms for challenging problems of the subject, often understood as 'private' and 'sensitive'.

In most Western cultures, the hardcore of mental illness traditionally associated with lunacy, madness, debility and other psychopathologies has transformed into a much wider set of emotional and social challenges and stigmatizing views have reduced in combination with the trivialization and the expansion of mental health culture. The current problems were mostly unrecognized as mental health issues in the 1950s or even in the 1970s in the context of work. The emotional or psychological hardships and symptoms were disguised as somatic problems, or they remained unrecognized or hidden.

The current understanding of mental vulnerability differs greatly from the pathological illness-driven understanding that was common 50 years ago. Today mental vulnerability is typically characterized by a tension between an active subject and the perception of poor opportunities to act in a meaningful way and according to one's own ideals. A psychologically alert subject takes care of their coping and makes use of information about the functioning of the psyche. Hence, a psychological working ability requires that the subject steps into the arena of mental health and pays attention to mental health in order to maintain their ability to work. From this point of view, vulnerability is part of the historical evolution of the subjectivity. At this point in history, examining one's emotions and recognizing psychological problems is reasonable. Both the vulnerable individual and the essence of vulnerability differ considerably from the notion of mental illness just a few decades ago.

In the current labour market, employees are expected to be flexible, adaptive and innovative (Boltanski and Chiapello, 2007; Varje et al, 2013a, 2013b). Social reality requires the ability to navigate in challenging and changing situations in an agile way. The emergence and proliferation of the entrepreneur-like character has produced a new demand for concepts such as mental health and wellbeing. When the human mind cannot handle fast pace, responsiveness and self-management, it has resulted in symptoms related to frustration, exhaustion and meaninglessness. The old approaches of occupational medicine and public health are not useful in this new reality, because the problems arise from emotional, interrelational and value-driven dimensions, and they are perceived and interpreted by historical subjects. In the treatment of the individual, psychological, therapeutic and psychopharmacological tools are increasingly used to take control over them (Lane, 2007; Illouz, 2008).

In a fast-cyclical economy emphasizing psychosocial dimensions and individualistic solutions, various arrangements (for example, recovery guidelines, short-term psychological consultancies) supporting mental work ability are promoted to reorganize the employees' psychological capacities and revitalize their mental fitness. In this context, analyses of wellness culture (Cederström and Spicer, 2015; Cabanas and Illouz, 2019; Ehrenreich, 2019) as well as psychopharmacology (Metzl, 2003; Jenkins, 2012; Brinkmann, 2016) have produced interesting observations. For example, they show how various agents of market economies benefit from the increasing broadening of mental health because their business logic is based on pastoral care and offering supporting services for help-seeking individuals (Salmenniemi, 2022: 5–6). From the point of view of the market economy, it is natural that demand creates services. At the same time, the economy of psychological support also produces new demand, which spreads through algorithms and social networks, for example.

Although cultural differences exist and there are specific dimensions of each political system affecting the behaviour of the population and mental vulnerabilities (Hofstede, 1980; Hall and Soskice, 2001; Amable, 2003; Sippola, 2012), mental health has become a part of how we understand work and occupational health in most affluent Western countries. Digitalization, intergenerational changes, the new emphasis on expert knowledge, individualization of behavioural strategies, the proliferation of information and service work and de-hierarchization of social relations are examples of these shared macro-level transitions that are common to most developed democratic countries. Psychological frameworks, entrepreneurial self-management and new mental health are examples of the consequences of this development. However, in different occupations and gendered working conditions the changes have partly differed, and they have treated population groups in different ways. At the same time, seen from a wider perspective of generations, work and occupational health, it is possible to outline some common underlying processes and several particular interrelationships behind the rise of mental vulnerability.

Parsing mental vulnerability in different disciplines

Sciences have had a significant role in the development of the phenomenon of mental vulnerability. The strengthening voice of the psycho-subjective field has progressed in society while the scientific disciplines have experienced a revolution. For example, health research has more clearly identified a world of new epidemiology susceptible to human influences that has become stronger alongside the world of exposures arising from biological, genetic and physical–chemical risks. In occupational health research and social epidemiology, the new world of exposure is typically labelled 'psychosocial' or 'socio-economic' risks leading to 'mental health outcomes' according to the natural science approach.

Already since the 1960s some social epidemiologists suggested that in the ensuing era of 'chronic disease risk factors' traditional epidemiology has come to an end, because further investigation of risks at the individual level will not lead to a comprehensive understanding of the birth of contemporary disease. For instance, a Southern African social epidemiologist, Mervyn Susser (1973), argued that states of health do not exist in a vacuum apart from people. People form societies, and any study of the attributes and health of people is also a study of the form, the structure and the processes of social forces. He called for the contribution of social sciences to epidemiology in the *Lancet* (Susser, 1964) and suggested an 'ecologic perspective' to public health researchers (Susser, 1973). This meant a rejection of the biology-driven paradigm and integration of social issues and experiences into the analysis of health transitions. The latter decades of the 20th century witnessed a considerable turn towards the 'social determinants' in the research of public health.

However, in public health explanatory models mainly turn to either individuals or structures, but the structure of individuals' actions is rarely grasped. What makes the situation challenging is the fact that many of the components and mechanisms affecting the structure of mental vulnerability cannot be measured with tools that measure individual conditions and circumstances as is done in traditional epidemiology and public health research. This also means that there is a need for reformation in the traditional public health and occupational health policy (Mercer, 2014: 217). In this book, I have tried to renew the research on the psyche of working-age people by bringing historical materials and social scientific perspectives into the analysis (Busfield, 2000: 551).

The perspective of historically changing agency and social character forms emphasizes three critical points in the study of mental vulnerability. First, outcomes and risks related to human behaviour take place in a certain historical context and their testing and detected associations do not provide a universal time-independent picture of the phenomenon. Second, work ability and socio-emotional health reflect the views, values and needs based on certain fitness criteria and work contexts. Due to the contextual nature of mental health and work ability, disability is related to changes in work and the subjectivity of the working individual. For this reason, the assessments and views concerning mental vulnerability are always located on the moving ground between culture, work and subjectivity. Third, the historicity of social existence frames the key questions and meaning of challenges for the subjects. The concepts and categories of the period influence the understanding and management of disability and the position of the psyche on the map of vulnerabilities.

Medical anthropologists have often made somewhat similar observations (Kleinman et al, 1985; Simons, 2003) as they emphasize the importance of culturally bound meaning making and social norms in defining and understanding health (Kleinman et al, 1978; Pike and Dunne, 2015). In turn, cross-cultural studies of mental health have indicated how Western psychosocial measures and subjective indicators of mental health do not necessarily capture the emotions and thoughts of people living in completely different circumstances and cultural value systems (for example, Kleinman et al, 1985; Marques, 2018; Ventevogel and Faiz, 2018). For instance, the somatization of emotional stress has been found to be more typical in many Asian cultures than in Western societies (Ryder et al, 2002).

Qualitative inquiries into different work cultures also provide highly relevant information on the importance of social structures of workplaces and the role of health and other social behaviours in distinctive organizational contexts. For example, in a factory in England studied by David Collinson (2010), the low and unstable social position of the workers led to counterculture and nonconformist behaviour at work. The workers found the managerial attempts to introduce humanist 'happy family' and 'team effort' concepts simply as derogative and responded to them with a variety of recalcitrant behaviours. Interestingly, most organizational problems and negative emotions were not intended to be resolved in the area of mental health (Collinson, 2010: 11). Finnish sociologist Matti Kortteinen (1992) has made partly similar observations in his studies on blue-collar machinists and white-collar bank clerks. He showed that the strategies used to resolve grievances in Finnish workplaces are very different in different occupations. The machinists relied on independence and resistance, while bank clerks intended to identify and get involved with the official goals and build their wellbeing by using official tools (see also Varje, 2018). These observations imply that class-related masculine work ethos and gendered organizational practices may even work as a counterculture against formal practices of mental health and organizational wellbeing. As described in Chapter 8, it is plausible that norms and codes of emotionality and organizational behaviours related to gender and occupation are likely to be reflected in the gender differences in the field of mental vulnerability.

The social history of work provides interesting material for rethinking mental vulnerabilities. For instance, the work by Peter Stearns (Stearns, 2010) and James Suzman (2021) as well as our studies have demonstrated how ideals concerning good workers and work ability are intertwined with valued citizenship and the role of work in social structure. Due to the complex historical relationship between work, subject and mental vulnerability, I am rather doubtful concerning the ideas regarding general impoverishment and increasing burdening of work. For instance, industrial 'modern work' is far too often interpreted as being impoverished, alienating and devoid of any meaning (Strangleman, 2007). The analyses of the present often disregard the active role of social agency and the needs for flexibility and mental capacities that were needed at work before our time (Gorz, 1999). Even though we talk about the 'golden age of work', the economic boom after the Second World War also had its problems related to long working hours and the status of women, for example. As the historical materials described also show, the transformation of work has changed the nature of work ability in practice and in sciences.

Labour market changes created new demands of capital and repositioned work ability. From the end of the 1900s, the employee ideals and requirements were increasingly connected to mental and social capacities necessary in service and information-based work organizations (Irvine, 2021: 3). From this perspective, it is not a surprise that scientific disciplines studying work and health have been increasingly concerned with mental health and psychological coping (Albrecht, 2015) and mental vulnerability has gained a new legitimacy as a research object.

Research combining observations from different disciplines of science calls for greater attention to questions of epistemology. As mental vulnerability is created in both social and biological arenas, we need *multiple* epistemologies since the assumptions we make with respect to the biological aspects of human existence do not necessarily hold for social behaviour (Newton, 2022). For example, approaches of social psychology studying work and wellbeing at work should parse individual forms of behaviour and group phenomena as part of a larger society and its cultural codes (Sullivan, 2020). This means that also methods need to be reconsidered. I believe that the dynamics of mental vulnerability can be traced and understood better by making use of different methods and materials such as observational, interview and documentary data (Flick, 2018; Hammersley and Atkinson, 2019; Bartholomew and Brown, 2022; Newton, 2022). In my opinion, research on vulnerability can also be diversified by utilizing more traditional surveys, health registers and new types of digital data sources that are constantly emerging. So, the use of multiple epistemologies also signifies the application of new research techniques as well.

It is essential to consider the impact of the scientific paradigm. The fundamental way mental health and work is viewed differs quite considerably if we apply interactional-constructivism versus policy-demography level realism paradigms as a framework of our analysis. In the former, 'mental health' is 'formed' and 'negotiated' while in the latter it is influenced by 'determinants' and 'factors'. Consequently, within these scientific paradigms quite distinctive views of the very nature of the subject matter are offered. One of the key questions behind this book has been how to build scientific knowledge about mental health and changing society. This makes us think about how valid and legitimate research information on work ability and mental health is formed, and how it contributes to the phenomenon it deals with in society (see Flick, 2018).

The philosopher Isaiah Berlin described the Greek fable of the hedgehog and the fox (Berlin, 1953), which has also been used for educational purposes in the sciences (for example, McKee et al, 2013). In the fable, the hedgehog knew one big thing, but the fox knew many little things, and this led to different worldviews. In the sciences of mental health and work, there is an ongoing controversy between grand unifying theories that would explain a phenomenon in its totality and between strategies of details searching for numerous different explanations, each explaining a specific detail of the phenomenon. Currently, most knowledge on mental vulnerability among the working-aged seems to be constructed by collecting information on limited details, like work demands, availability of mental health services, income level, personality or economic cycles. Especially in the media, these discoveries are repeatedly framed as if these details have somehow proved that there are some sort of ironbound laws surrounding mental health and disorders. However, perhaps the fox should try to see broader transitions in the foundations, circumstances and concepts of behaviour, and perhaps the hedgehog should look into the local and sometimes paradoxical details.

One of the main themes of this book has been the role of the subject / social agency in the study of mental health and work. In Western traditions, the 'self' or 'subjectivity' is typically considered a reflexive concept that refers to processes that happen 'internally', that is, within the person, while dialogue typically takes place 'externally', that is, between the person and the other (Tafarodi, 2013: 4). This model of thinking has guided thinking about work and mental health towards the direction of seeing the individual and their environment as separate entities that influence each other. Cultural norms, conceptual frames of reference or institutional possibilities that affect the individual's self and social subjectivity have not been analysed. In this book, I have tried to merge the analysis of the exogenous conditions and subjectivity by using the analytical categories of 'social character' and 'mental vulnerability'. When mental vulnerability is considered as a changing phenomenon linked to relationships and production requirements, connections to occupational class, gender and other contextual frameworks and possibilities of the activity emerge (Eaton et al, 2010). This also highlights the historical nature of vulnerability. For example, exhaustion did not play the same role in the pre-industrial labour market as it does today, because the understanding of mental health problems was different then and mental illness was not recognized as a health challenge in the same way as it is now (for example, Schaffner, 2017). A healthy body was considered a prerequisite for mental wellbeing, but mental ability to work was not an end in itself.

Various disciplines and expert knowledge based on them played an important role in identifying mental health and raised social awareness of the possibility of vulnerability. During the past decades the sciences that have studied the expanding mental health field have offered new perspectives, classifications and expert roles and moved the old-fashioned narrow mental illness and patient-oriented approach to the margins. As societies change, the field that studies mental health and work has also diversified, but individual-level perspectives have remained persistently strong. The social actor that changes with society has remained mainly a silent figure in mental health research. It has also had an impact on how the psychological and social problems of working people have been perceived and the ways in which scientific knowledge has been used to capture them. In mainstream occupational health and wellbeing research, the essence of people has been seen as relatively unchanged, even though changes in the economy and culture have produced a new kind of social structure in which vulnerability is being framed and rebuilt.

Wellness medicine

A periodization of medicine developed by medical sociologist David Armstrong (1995; see also Ackerknecht, 1967) on the 'spatialization of illness' over the centuries in Western countries provides important insights on the changing social position of medicine in relation to mental vulnerability (see Foucault, 1973). In the earlier period of modernity, the clinician's task in 'bedside medicine' was to identify and classify illness through the distinctiveness of clusters of symptoms. Hospitals did not exist, and patient were taken care of at home. The mobility of illness through the body tried to be captured by closely monitoring the sequence of symptoms and going systematically through patients' experiences. This period was followed by 'hospital medicine', where the physician's job changed to examining the patient's body by using clinical examination and inferring the underlying pathological lesion. In consequence, for the first time, the biological processes of the patient's body became the focus of medical attention. Many techniques of clinical examination developed. The stethoscope, X-rays and blood tests are examples of the development of hospital medicine (Armstrong, 1995). Hospital medicine often required the neutral space of the hospital or a clinic so that the indicators of the underlying lesion could be detected and treated.

Based on a myriad of observations presented in this book, I propose that at the end of the 20th and the beginning of the 21st century we have witnessed a growth of a new type of medical practice that has risen next to hospital medicine. In 'wellness medicine' active patients interact with doctors and other professionals, use consulting services and digital channels. The relationship is less hierarchical and more reciprocal than in earlier phases of medicine (McKinlay and Marceau, 2002; Elston, 2009). In this behavioural setting doctors use a shared decision-making model based on interaction and considering the patient's opinion (Renedo et al, 2018). In wellness medicine, patients have become clients who pay attention to their emotional wellbeing and mental coping. Under this new model of action, both professionals and non-professionals are alert to observe, report and act upon potential threats.

The shift towards wellness medicine is related to the transformation of the behaviour of the social character and the standards of mental health. Feelings and thoughts arising from, among other things, work challenges are increasingly being channelled to be treated by wellness medicine. At the same time, the 'moving target' of mental health has resettled into a new place. Although mental health problem still carries a negative stigma to some extent, the range of symptoms and cases that drift into the area of healthcare has grown strongly since the late 20th century. Mental health has merged with diverse themes related to the management of life and work, which applies to practically anyone. Historically, it is evident that the change in the code of social behaviour and the structural changes in the production of capital have moved the health professionals working with the active workforce, such as occupational health doctors and nurses, increasingly into the non-clinical area of wellness management.

The findings of our research (Väänänen et al, 2019; Wilkinson and Väänänen, 2021) suggest that in the late 1900s and early 2000s, the reconfiguration of the social relationships between the occupational health professionals and patients served to create social opportunities and spaces for doctors taking care of employees to be more attentive to clients' experiences of emotional distress. In this way, wellness medicine developed gradually as working conditions, organizational changes and employees' life challenges began to be treated in the formal system of health and disability. The democratization of the clinical encounter facilitated a more open and fulsome expression of emotional discontent. At the same time, the medicalization of mental health continued as demands for new treatments were recognized and the pressure to capture individuals' emotional distress increased.

One of the main tensions within the context of wellness medicine is between subjective non-material and organic/observable work ability. This is related to the paradox between health and work ability; although the external frameworks of wellbeing and the possibilities of treating organic health problems of the population have considerably improved, anxiety, depression, exhaustion, attention deficit hyperactivity disorder and other conditions related to the management and recalibration of social and emotional behaviour have increased. In medical care, Google-based diagnostics and looking for second opinions have accompanied this change. Wellness medicine intends to solve the challenge of subjective suffering and discomfort by developing new psychological measures and more effective interactive strategies. At the same time, psychiatric nurses, psychologists and other professionals who are trained to support the clients' psyche have integrated in the treatment of new vulnerabilities (Barling and Griffiths, 2003; Wilkinson and Väänänen, 2021).

American historian of medicine Charles Rosenberg (1992) has analysed the changing nature of mental health using the concept of the 'social framing' of illness. Both doctors and their clients create a picture of the phenomenon and its features using collectively shared criteria and classification systems that 'frame' the phenomenon called mental health. However, Rosenberg's approach does not mean that the challenges of the mind do not exist or do not have a material basis. Rather, he emphasizes how the psyche is always understood, interpreted and treated through certain views, institutions and roles that change over time. Philosophically, his theoretical view approaches critical realism (Bhaskar, 1998), which recognizes the importance of social changes in the development of concepts and categories (Wilkinson, 2017; see also Figert, 1996). The concept of 'framing' helps to structure the consequences of expert knowledge on the micro level of behaviour. As scientific knowledge changes, people's perceptions of work ability change and, as a result, their behaviour also changes.

Similarly, cultural researchers of health have observed that illness categories can affect people's experiences of being sick, and over time people learn to be sick in an accepted way (Kleinman et al, 1978: 252; Bröer and Besseling, 2017). This perspective differs from social constructionism, emphasizing the discursive and negotiated nature of mental health, which easily generates negative and hostile attitudes among employees and their families, who easily feel that this kind of interpretation denies the pain and suffering involved in mental health challenges (Busfield, 2000). In this context, it is important to note that this book's historical analysis does not imply a critique of the actions of individuals or employees or an understatement of their experiences. Nor does it seek to deny the genuine benefits of the work of skilled psychologists and other psychological support professionals in clients' lives. Rather, I have tried to understand the phenomenon of mental vulnerability from the perspective of changing societal frameworks. After all, the socio-cultural change has affected – and affects – the entire population almost without exception.

Rosenberg's (2006) analysis of the position of psychiatry is also interesting. He suggests that during the 20th century, psychiatry did little to address the social status and growth of multiplied psychiatric disease categories in the classification of new populations. According to him, by focusing on somatics and turning to pharmacological solutions, psychiatry has tried to increase its legitimacy in the medical field. Psychiatry has been dominated by 'rationalization forces' that aim to reduce health problems to specific causes and treatments (Kleinman and Becker, 1998; Rosenberg, 2006). As a result, there have been many contradictions and conflicts within the scientific field and many researchers have started to analyse the cultural characteristics of mental wellbeing and illness.

Interestingly, the typical forms of mental vulnerability in current work are treated relatively little in psychiatry. Psychiatry mainly treats patients who have struggled with serious mental health challenges often for a long time. In the work of occupational health physicians and occupational health care in general, support for ordinary employees in their everyday lives and coping at work is increasingly emphasized. In this way, wellness medicine highlights ordinary life and the possibility for anyone to need support. In other words, the emphasis is on helping the customer as an employee and productive citizen.

It seems that the transition of societal conditions and population behaviour have especially influenced the branches of medicine which take care of people in their mundane contexts. The work of occupational health doctors reflects this kind of treatment of the psyche intimately linked to the structure of production and the social context. Within occupational medicine, societal change is penetrating into medicine in new forms of behaviour and conversation. The change has created a need for new approaches. In our own interviews occupational health doctors told how descriptive diagnoses related to various emotional and mental problems have become more common in their work. As medical experts, doctors also contested the 'advancements'. Many of the observed changes in mental health problems were viewed as definitional. They were also critical about the emergence of ever-increasing diagnostic categories (American Psychiatric Association, 2013; WHO, 2014). Efforts have been made to take control of the changing situation in the work of doctors by developing screening tools, questionnaires and good practices to evaluate, measure and treat mental health.

The current wellness medicine had a pre-history in public health research, for example, before its final emergence. The examples of the broadening of mental health started to emerge already at the beginning in the 1950s when the 'social indicators movement' initiated studying the 'quality of life' with a focus on how it varied by population groups and how it changes (Land, 1975; Andrews and Withey, 1976). Researchers of applied psychology also began to pay attention to the wellbeing of citizens and workplaces, especially since the 1970s. Concepts such as satisfaction, happiness and the recognition of human potential began to be seen as valid research topics (Neugarten, 1973; Diener et al, 1999; Seligman and Csikszentmihalyi, 2000; Manderscheid et al, 2010; Ryff and Singer, 2013). In this way, the brief history of wellness medicine is strongly related to the birth of the health promotion paradigm that aims to develop the wellbeing of the entire population.

While mental wellbeing became a cultural value, the recognition of the importance of the emotional experience of the subject paved the way for a new language and new channels for expressing both distress and wellbeing. The observations suggest that the position of mental health oriented to wellbeing began to expand when the importance of rigid class structures and social hierarchies decreased in society. Cultural liberation and the growth of social reformism influenced the birth of radical psychiatry, public health research and humanistic psychology. With the cultural change, the sciences that study the psyche began to change and involve new contents, as the researchers began to consider and emphasize the views of individuals and employees from different social backgrounds. One dimension of this transition was the research of the quality of work and wellbeing at work. Frederick Herzberg, Arthur Kornhauser, David Katz, Einar Thursrud, Bertil Gardell, Lennart Levi and many others started to study psychological wellbeing in the workplace in a new way. Their research emphasized developing psychological conditions that produce wellbeing (Väänänen et al, 2012).

Today various arguments promoting mental health propose that mental health issues are like any other health problems and should be dealt as such – within the context of adequate health prevention and healthcare. However, the dramatic spread of mental health disabilities and worries in society raise doubts about how contemporary mental health approaches work. It seems reasonable to ask whether recognition and prevention have started to produce manifestations of vulnerability, which should be treated outside healthcare and the framework of health. Or to what extent the increased services and conceptual frameworks of wellness medicine produce a mental health culture without borders, and identities that conform to it?

Mental health as a ritual

According to several analyses, disability is closely connected to adult identity in a society based on the norms of work and good workership (Niemi and Mietola, 2017; Hakala et al, 2018). The role of work in the formation of citizenship has been important throughout modern history. For example, the American theology of success in the 1900s was based on the influence of Protestantism. Earthly success was seen as a sign of God's love and being on the right moral path. This meant that the worker's ideals were often seamlessly aligned with the theological and economic mission. Today's mental health theology, in turn, involves more psychological self-care and the intentions to search for a direction loyal to oneself. Instead of priests, the current support more involves personal trainers, wellness consultants and therapists. Even the new supportive functions of the church have moved towards therapeutic means and psychological consultation. From the perspective of the employees, the secularization and individualization of the soul have meant new models and structures of behaviour built around subjective mental wellbeing.

The analysis of the 'techniques of the body' developed by French sociologist and social anthropologist Marcel Mauss (1973 [1934]) offers us an interesting perspective that might help to understand the social dynamics of mental vulnerability in our culture. Mauss described techniques of the body as highly automatized actions that embody aspects and influences of the surrounding culture. They can differ according to class, gender and other social background characteristics. For instance, the manners of eating, practising sports and wearing clothes have differed according to historical time and social position. In his study, Mauss himself applied cross-national differences in techniques such as digging and walking that he had observed during the First World War as an example. He emphasized that all the elements of action are dominated by the facts of cultural education. According to Mauss's theorizing, most everyday actions have been learnt and are based on a shared understanding of appropriate styles and manners and modes of acting. He called them 'techniques'.

Applying Mauss's theory, we can think that employees use different techniques when confronted with a mentally difficult situation at work or in their personal life. They are learnt and socially shared. For example, coping strategies for work stress and other psychologically challenging situations suggested by organizational consultants and work ability specialists are examples of the techniques that we are offered. They can include, for example, time management or mindfulness. Revitalizing depleted psychological and biochemical resources is thought to best happen by learning body-mind techniques that shield the mind. Their large-scale application can influence the solution models that are seen as appropriate ways to solve problems related to distress at work, for example.

If we continue with the social anthropological interpretation, mental vulnerabilities seem to carry several ritualistic features (Bericat, 2016). Like rituals in general, rituals related to mental health encapsulate the priorities and goals of a community. They generate group emotions and create a base for a shared culture (Summers-Effler, 2006: 135). In traditional communities, rituals were performed in social gatherings in which individuals maintained the same focus of attention, shared the same values and felt the same emotions (Knottnerus, 2010; Bericat, 2016). Taking the sacrificial rituals of aboriginal Australians as an example, Durkheim (1965 [1912]) described the basic mechanisms through which collective events produced and maintained the social cohesion of the group (Bericat, 2016).

Today, there are rituals related to nurturing and improving mental health, which are promoted and built in different communities devoted to the matter. They collectively share values and goals that have to do with mental health. Organizational developers, stakeholders, advocacy communities and researchers are active participants in producing techniques meant for supporting work ability in their own communities in the sake of strengthening mental health. In the culture of mental health, occupational groups and citizens have a multitude of social media forums where information and views of the best possible mental health practices are described and promoted.

Techniques and rituals of mental health are so widely spread that they are hard to see. For example, guidebooks, expert-interview articles and blogposts produce material for rituals. The expressions 'healthy workplaces' and 'sustainable industries' engage these rituals. Different networking events and webinars offer space for sharing experiences and views (Turner, 1969; Murray, 1989). Responsible supervisors understand the importance of good mental health for the work community and job performance and encourage paying attention to psychological well-being. Rituals are used in a variety of situations and they have a social function: to tackle the mental health crisis and make the necessary investments as soon as possible before it is too late.

The population is increasingly interested in the development of various behavioural techniques of mental health. As a concrete indication of the growing role of techniques of mental health, the number of people using state-subsidized psychotherapy grew from 15,000 to more than 60,000 in Finland in 2011–2021 due to cultural and legislation changes, while in the early 2000s this was fewer than 10,000 people (Social Security Institution of Finland, 2022b). Today mental health has become strongly politicized and it is constantly used as a reason for different recommendations and interventions. For instance, speedy and timely access to mental health services has been very popular topic in the political debate in Finland during recent years. The spread of mental health rituals can be explained by today's societies' need to maintain a 'moral society'. Anthropologist Roy Rappaport (1999), a pioneer in ritual research, sees this as the basic purpose of rituals. It is plausible that mental health practices provide us with a 'moral approach' to deal with difficult and community-threatening issues that would otherwise be difficult to deal with collectively.

Rituals call for specific techniques. From the perspective of the subject, this idea of techniques is closely connected to Michel Foucault's (1988) idea of the 'practices of the self' through which the subject constitutes itself in the community (see Kelly, 2013). With the practices of the self, the subject finds different modes of action in his culture and, at the same time, they are proposed or imposed upon him by his culture and his social group (Foucault, 1984: 291; Kelly, 2013). Rituals can be seen as a central way in which techniques are shared from one individual or group to another. They are social behaviours that often have some shared ethical purpose. According to Foucault, ethics can be seen as the elaboration of self that enables an individual to fashion themself into a subject of ethical conduct in their community (Foucault, 1984: 263). Thus, ethics is defined by Foucault as one way for people to constitute themselves as subjects. Ethics is not a matter of rules or principles for actions that can be labelled as 'right' or 'good', 'ethical' or 'moral', but rather it is part of the formation of the social character in each society (Kelly, 2013). The prevailing ethical practices, or in Mauss's terms, techniques, suggest ways of working that we should use to take care of ourselves and develop ourselves towards 'the best version of me'.

From the perspective of the individual, the present ethic of mental vulnerability at work can be summed up in two practices:

1. We should take care of ourselves as well as we can.
2. We should intend to know ourselves so that we can tolerate the effects produced by work and other challenges.

Nowadays, for instance, wearable digital devices are used for self-monitoring one's own behaviour and bodily states (Lupton, 2016). Sport trackers and sleep monitors are examples of devices that are designed to help people to take care of themselves. The use of these techniques is often justified by arguments derived from the field of wellness medicine and mental health.

With institutionalized practices, challenges ranging from the macro-level (for example, productivity demands), meso-level (for example, lack of organized work process) or individual level (for example, abilities) are easily transformed to the vocabularies and techniques of mental health. In *mental healthification* (on healthification, see Fusco, 2006), the problems of everyday life are intended to be solved by transferring burdening challenges into the fields of individual self-care, treatment and recovery. From this perspective, it is less surprising that sickness absences related to psychiatric reasons, psychotropic medication and mental-illness-related rehabilitation underwent a steep rise in the 2000s and 2010s, even though work disability due to somatic problems diminished. As different challenges of work and the burdens of life have become 'mental healthified' at the individual level, they have increasingly become public health and disability concerns at the population level. This can be seen, for instance, in the debate on the effectiveness of antidepressants and continuous discussion on mental health policies. If we go two or three generations back, we do not detect these techniques, rituals or ethics at almost any level of the society.

It has been proposed that, currently, mental health is one of the key 'languages of suffering' in everyday life (Brinkmann, 2016). Within this cultural context, older generations sometimes feel confused in the face of growing mental health problems among young people. New rituals and practices related to mental healthification may be difficult to understand for people who have grown up in an environment of different ethical norms and standards of health. Rituals, vocabularies and identities related to mental healthification are more widely recognized and shared among the generations of welfare and therapy culture. The status of subjective wellbeing and emotions is associated with the new ethics of behaviour and older generations have difficulties seeing where are the borders and what to think about the situation.

However, it is important to note that according to our research materials the perceptions of mental health and its status differ even within the same generation of young adults. Not all groups are equally attached to mental health rituals. There are also differences between those who look at working life from different perspectives. For instance, the ideas of challenged wellbeing at work promoted by organizational consultants and human resources management often differ from employees' experiences and emphasis. At the grassroots level, the approaches proposed by consultants and specialists may seem external and may even backfire. This can appear, for example, in the form of sarcasm in the workplace. This means that views on mental heathification include tensions and contradictions in the work cultures and society at large. Rituals are not uniform either, but contain different standings, emphases and preferences.

Although crisis talk concerning mental health often describes the intensity and specificity of the current situation, it can be justly argued we have been on this track for several decades now. Unlike in past centuries, the gaze of an increasing part of the population has been directed towards meaningful life goals and feelings of personal satisfaction. Work sociologist Marc Loriol (2019; 184–185) summarizes that today, for instance, work is expected to be 'useful' in accordance with certain personal criteria. Work should offer opportunities for learning, development, autonomy and feelings of meaningfulness. Some scholars, such as Daniel Bell, have interpreted such findings as an indication of the wider spread of a culture of hedonism and pleasure to the area of work (Bell, 1996).

This has to do with the development of a culture based on emotions. Some researchers who have studied the change of the emotional culture have proposed that in the current mundane life, we witness countless discussions on what different feelings mean, and 'we are constituted by our emotions and feelings' (McCarthy, 2002). Mental vulnerability can be added to the equation by the fact that the negotiation of the boundaries of late modern work and everyday life often causes feelings of dissatisfaction and confusion. Lack of time and other key resources dampen the idealism related to development and personal meaningfulness. This increases the likelihood of entering the area of different feelings of scarcity as well as the arenas of mental health rituals.

From the perspective of institutions and politics, the interest and political influence related to expanded mental health has started to resemble a social movement (Tilly, 2004; Alapuro, 2018), where the goals of various interest groups, the views of experts and the utilitarianism of commercial agents are intersected and sometimes collide. The movement can be seen in many aspects of work culture, such as occupational safety guidelines, psychological occupational safety legislation, and themes raised by trade unions. In a society sensitized to mental vulnerability, various actors in the mental health field offer views and ideas on how to understand and name the challenge, how to treat it, how to position it in relation to other social problems and how to use this perspective to identify oneself and other people. In this way, mental health has also been linked in a new way to the exercise of power in the labour market. Consequently, the multi-vocal mental health movement touches millions of employees, professionals, advocacy groups and decision-makers. This cultural fabric includes a large number of procedures, information structures and techniques attached to the topic.

In current societies, mental health plays many social roles. It is ethical self-listening, risk prevention, emotional processing, maintaining work ability, securing livelihoods and so on. Challenges related to abilities, social conflicts, work–family conflicts, personal goals as well as various social areas of life are increasingly attached to the potential vulnerability of the mind and the risk of deteriorating work ability. The strong legitimacy of the health paradigm ('healthism') directs the solution of problems towards a culturally valued treatment and diagnostic framework. In health forums, the vulnerable psyche gets a specific status and importance. It turns into symptom descriptions, measurements and often medical diagnoses. It becomes a medical and psychological fact that should be treated individually. Cynicism, fatigue, melancholy and other human experiences are being mental-healthified and moved towards wellness medicine.

At the beginning of this book, I started with sociologist David Riesman and colleagues (1950), whose analytical framework on the change of the social character is interesting. In the mid-1900s they analysed the societal transition in the United States, suggesting that during the period of modernization and urbanization Americans moved towards an 'other-directedness', which has been associated with an increase in openness, empathy and tolerance, 'a more humane and accommodating responsiveness' between people. Partly in a similar way, Norbert Elias (1991) emphasized that the advancing division of labour and growth of communities required the transformation of external controls into the subjects' internal controls to properly function in extensive chains of interaction (Shilling and Mellor, 2022). Other-directed behaviour has been increasingly demanded and made possible by 'pressures operating upon the individual' (Elias, 1991: 374).

In the light of many examples from the labour market, it seems obvious that system-based (for example, expert work, production chains) and interactional (for example, service and knowledge work) demands related to the advancement of modernity are evidently present in the advancement of mental vulnerability. Emotional pressures have advanced within modern organizations in which flexibility, psychosocial abilities and managing one's own emotions has been considered a fundamental asset. But at the same time, it is also about the historical change of the human control system, where the role of subjective experience (mental wellbeing, emotional satisfaction, and so on) has become central in determining the direction of behaviour.

Changes in work towards intangible services and information and a fundamental shift towards emotion management systems emphasizing the weight of the individual's psyche have strengthened the tendency that some social scientists have called 'overheating' (Ziehe, 1991; Eriksen, 2016). This book has dealt with this multigenerational change and its side effects from the point of view of mental health and work. On the other hand, it has also shown opposite trends, which could be called 'cooling off'. In these cases, themes of psychological vulnerability have started to emerge, for example, when certain professional skills have lost their value due to changes in work processes, or when one's work input is only occasionally needed in the labour market. Whatever it is, the matter has increasingly moved into the area of mental health and individual wellness management.

From the perspective of the history of ideas today, we go through the effects produced by many historical layers. The ideals of the Age of Enlightenment, from human orientation to emphasizing the status of scientific knowledge, can be seen as threads in current social activities and ideals. The emphasis on the importance of emotions of the Romantic era, in turn, echoes the themes of self-listening and self-exploration (Lupton, 1998). Mental vulnerability also reflects the 1960s politics of human rights and the discourses of psychological humanism. The spread of mental health became possible when equality, freedom of expression and self-development became more firmly connected to modern humanity. In this context of cultural history, one can also observe an intensification of approaches and concepts, in which the specificity of the human individual in relation to the rest of the surrounding world is emphasized.

From the ecological perspective, the natural scientists Paul Crutzen and Eugene Stoermer (for example, Crutzen, 2000) proposed naming the current geological era the Anthropocene, based on the realization that human footprints can be seen everywhere on the planet. According to the themes raised in this book, the transition towards the age of Anthropocene is not only changing our planet, but it has considerably changed ourselves and our social being. From the perspective of mental vulnerabilities, the perspective of the Anthropocene directs our attention towards institutions, ideologies and social practices focused on humans and their wellbeing. It seems evident that we have started to focus more on human resources, social relationships between humans, psychological aspects and mental health issues.

The human-centred ethics and goals described have received widespread support. However, it is possible to see that the increase in the value of subjective human experience has also led to partly unpredictable developments. For example, the background of the mental health crisis is probably a long-continued development, where listening and evaluating the mental state of new population groups has become the centre of cultural morality. It rears its head in repeated speeches that emphasize consideration of human resources or the importance of psychological wellbeing. Human experience is everywhere, and it is used to justify decisions and actions everywhere (MacCormack, 2020; see also Braidotti, 2019: 62–63). Since mental health is at the core of late modern humanity, we can think that while we study the emergence of mental vulnerability and its forms, mechanisms and consequences, we also study the humanization of Western work culture and society. From this point of view, it can be thought that the growth of the role of mental health in production and the working population is largely a by-product of the same social and economic process as the climate crisis.

Since mental health is about people and their wellbeing, it is possible that we are dealing with the crisis of a cultural way of thinking that focuses on people and human communities by looking at problem areas like mental health. In this sense, the status of mental health is a symptom of a society that has turned with considerable force to the subjective experience of humans. In terms of the health and wellbeing of the working-age population, it is a radical historical change. Both the labour market and the employee themselves have started to deal with the problems of the subjective world through emotional wellbeing, mental work capacity and psychological approaches. Late modern individualization and the relaxation of power relations have thus opened the way for processing of emotions and psychological states in immeasurable amounts. At the same time, completely new fields of activity and social agency positions have emerged, where human experience is reflected and aimed at steering in a favourable direction.

I have personally found Michel Foucault's (2005, [1966]) depiction of disappearing traces on a sandy beach in *The Order of the Things* illuminating. In that passage, he reflected on the historically changing and disappearing nature of knowledge: how the knowledge of human nature transforms, and how we as humans are historically conditional. I think it is likely that recently emerged practices and frameworks concerning mental health will gradually vanish, and new approaches will appear. With the advent of change, outdated patterns and rituals are masked by new points of uneasiness, ability ideals, health perceptions, and ways of dealing with problems in social and emotional life. In the coming moment of history, researchers dealing with our period may ask how we, as builders of knowledge and professionals of the early 2000s, ended up with such problems, and attempted to find solutions in an area that we called 'work and mental health'.

Original publications of the research group

Table A.1: Original publications of the research group

Name	Aim	Material	Method	Theory	Main findings
Väänänen, A., Murray, M. and Kuokkanen, A. (2014). The growth and the stagnation of work stress: Publication trends and scientific representations 1960–2011. *History of the Human Sciences*, 27(4), 116–138. https://doi.org/10.1177/0952695114525168	To examine secular trends in scientific publications on work stress, and analyse how, over a period of 50 years, a new discursive, institutional, intellectual and subjective space of work stress has developed.	Scientific articles on work stress in three major databases and 12 well-established journals from 1960 to 2011.	Quantitative analysis of secular trends in work stress publications and qualitative critical analysis of a smaller sample of work stress publications (N=132).	Theory of social representations, critical theories of science and historical sociology of occupational health.	The number of work stress publications rose steeply until the early 2000s and the growth evened out and even started to decline in some sources in the early 2010s. The development of scientific representations of work stress can be understood as an integral part of the larger social, cultural and economic shift that has required novel approaches and management methods. As one of the key life-structuring representations of the late 20th century and the early 21st century 'work stress' absorbed various unpleasant characteristics of late modern work.
Väänänen, A., Anttila, E., Turtiainen, J. and Varje, P. (2012). Formulation of work stress in 1960–2000: Analysis of scientific works from the perspective of historical sociology. *Social Science & Medicine*, 75(5), 784–795. https://doi.org/10.1016/j.socscimed.2012.04.014	To examine the process of formulating and defining the concept of work stress in the occupational health sciences and in industrial and organizational psychology between 1960 and 2000.	107 scientific articles, books, book chapters, 'state-of-the-art' reviews, book reviews, and written conference presentations.	The approach of 'anthropology of knowledge', concentrating on the intellectual life of scientific groups, circles and 'epistemological communities'.	The frameworks of historical sociology, critical psychology and the anthropology of knowledge.	Work stress as a life-structuring concept gained ground in various scientific communities in the 1960s simultaneously with the rise of social reformist movements emphasizing human-orientated work organizations and socially responsible values. With the passing of time, however, the focus on structural improvement of work life waned and the emphasis shifted towards the apolitical occupational health aspects of work stress.

(continued)

Table A.1: Original publications of the research group (continued)

Name	Aim	Material	Method	Theory	Main findings
Varje, P. and Väänänen, A. (2016). Health risks, social relations and class: An analysis of occupational health discourse in Finnish newspaper and women's magazine articles 1961–2008. *Sociology of Health & Illness*, 38(3), 493–510. https://doi.org/10.1111/1467-9566.12376	To investigate how class expectations have been linked with the redefinition of occupational health risks during the period 1961–2008.	Occupational-health-related articles in the Finnish newspaper *Helsingin Sanomat* (HS), and the women's magazine *Me Naiset* (MN) from 1961 to 2008.	Analysis of historical textual materials and discourse analysis.	Historical sociology, social class theories and critical theories.	After the 1970s, social relations at the workplace became problematized and the image of the hierarchical organization was replaced by idealized middle-class notions. The public discussion has been shaped by a collision between the dominant middle-class expectations of harmony and equality and the neoliberal production of competition and inequality.
Väänänen, A., Turtiainen, P., Kuokkanen, A. and Petersen, A. (2019) From silence to diagnosis: The entry of the mentally problematic employee into medical practice. *Social Theory & Health*, 17(4), 407–426. https://doi.org/10.1057/s41285-019-00101-4	To explore how occupational health physicians perceive the changes that have enabled the emergence of mental health concerns in the Finnish welfare regime.	41 in-depth interviews of occupational health professionals with a long career. Most of them had worked from the 1970s to the 2000s.	In-depth interviews and critical content analysis of the material collected.	History-informed theories: informalization, democratization and medicalization.	The results emphasize three historical transformations: (1) the loosening of the stigma related to mental health problems (informalization of mental health problems); (2) the changing character of employees/patients (psychologically aware customers); and (3) the paradox of a new medical culture (decreasing medical dominance and increasing medicalization).
Wilkinson, I. and Väänänen, A. (2021). The informalization of doctor–patient relations in a Finnish setting: New social figurations and emergent possibilities. *Sociology of Health & Illness*, 43(9), 1965–1980. https://doi.org/10.1111/1467-9566.13375	To explore the value of an Eliasian approach towards interpreting and assessing the moral meanings and social dynamics of relationships between health practitioners and their patients.	41 in-depth interviews of occupational health professionals with a long career. Most of them had worked from the 1970s to the 2000s.	In-depth interviews with health professionals and theory-driven analysis of the collected material.	Norbert Elias's theory on spiralling formalizing and informalizing processes.	Finnish occupational health professionals made efforts to renegotiate social roles, cultural meanings and individual responsibilities. This can be taken as an instance where informalization is accompanied by revitalized currents of formalization and new syntheses of moral codes and conduct. The results describe how mental health is negotiated within historically specific work and health frameworks.

Table A.1: Original publications of the research group (continued)

Name	Aim	Material	Method	Theory	Main findings
Kuokkanen, A., Varje, P. and Väänänen, A. (2020). Struggle over employees' psychological well-being: The politization and depolitization of the debate on employee mental health in the Finnish insurance sector. *Management & Organizational History*, 15(3), 252–272. https://doi.org/10.1080/17449359.2020.1845741	To examine the emergence and evolution of the discourse on mental health problems as an occupational health risk in the professional debates among Finnish insurance workers from a historical perspective.	Articles from *Kenttämies* and *Pasma*, the two company magazines of a Finnish insurance company, Pohjola, from 1955 to 2007, and *Vakuutusväki*, the magazine of the trade union of Finnish insurance workers, from 1955 to 2014.	Collecting archival material, discourse analysis of journal texts.	Theories of the emergence of the neoliberal labour market and theories of individualization.	The workplace democratization movement of the 1970s and the increasing power of trade unions paved the way for the recognition and manifestation of employees' mental ill-health. In the 1990s and 2000s the individualization trend led to the view that employees themselves were responsible for maintaining their mental health, limiting their opportunities to express their grievances at the workplace.
Anttila, E. and Väänänen, A. (2013). Rural schoolteachers and the pressures of community life: Local and cosmopolitan coping strategies in mid-twentieth-century Finland. *History of Education*, 42(2), 182–203. https://doi.org/10.1080/0046760X.2013.766267	To investigate rural schoolteachers' relationships with local village communities in mid-20th-century Finland.	Articles that were published in the Finnish elementary schoolteachers' weekly professional journal *Opettajain Lehti* from the period 1937–1939 and 1948–1950.	Archival study and analysis of collected articles.	Robert K. Merton's categories of 'local' and 'cosmopolitan' coping strategies.	The local strategy required that teachers adapt themselves to the social demands of community life, whereas the cosmopolitan strategy was manifested in the teachers' efforts to distance themselves from the local community. This reflected the professionalization of Finnish schoolteachers as well as a general social transition in which traditional community ties were gradually replaced by modern individualism.

(continued)

Table A.1: Original publications of the research group (continued)

Name	Aim	Material	Method	Theory	Main findings
Anttila, E. and Väänänen, A. (2015). From authority figure to emotion worker: Attitudes towards school discipline in Finnish schoolteachers' journals from the 1950s to the 1980s. *Pedagogy, Culture & Society*, 23(4), 555–574. https://doi.org/10.1080/14681366.2015.1015153	To analyse the change in attitudes towards school discipline in Finnish schoolteachers' professional journals from the late 1950s to the early 1980s.	Articles in *Opettajain lehti* at three points of time: in 1959–1960, 1969–1970 and 1979–1980.	Archival study and analysis of the collected articles.	Informalization by Cas Wouters.	At the beginning of the studied period, the discussions in the journals were dominated by conservative views, which promoted authoritarian solutions. Over the next decades, these discussions came to be dominated by progressive views, which placed great value on the individual needs and rights of children. This emphasized the nature of teaching as a form of emotional labour.
Anttila, E., Turtiainen, J., Varje, P. and Väänänen, A. (2018). Emotional labour in a school of individuals. *Pedagogy, Culture & Society*, 26(2), 215–231. https://doi.org/10.1080/14681366.2017.1378708	To examine Finnish discussions on student-centred school culture and teachers' emotional labour from a sociological and historical perspective.	Articles published in a Finnish teachers' professional magazine from 1979 to 2011.	Archival study and thematic analysis.	Emotional labour research and Wouters's studies on permissive culture.	Student-centred deals stayed dominant in Finnish schoolteachers' professional discussions. The emotional stress involved in student-centred teaching evoked criticism from teachers. Attitudes varied regarding the solutions to teacher stress. Some of the solutions emphasized improving teachers' emotional competence, whereas others centred on decreasing the amount of emotional labour.
Turtiainen, J., Anttila, E. and Väänänen, A. (2022). Social work, emotion management and the transformation of the welfare state. *Journal of Social Work*, 22(1), 68–86. https://doi.org/10.1177/1468017320973586	To analyse historically how external pressures and efficiency requirements jeopardize employees' ability to carry out emotional labour in the public sector.	Finnish social workers' accounts published in a professional trade paper in 1975–2009.	Archival study and theory-driven analysis of materials.	Emotional management by Sharon Bolton.	Social workers' emotional job requirements are embedded in and influenced by the broader social context. Workers' emotion management underwent changes and readjustments from the heyday of the expansive welfare state of the mid-1970s, through the severe economic recession of the 1990s, and was bound by the ideological reform of the Finnish welfare policy in the 1990s and 2000s.

Table A.1: Original publications of the research group (continued)

Name	Aim	Material	Method	Theory	Main findings
Turtiainen, J., Väänänen, A. and Varje, P. (2018). The pressure of objectives and reality: Social workers' perceptions of their occupational complexities in a trade journal in 1958–1999. *Qualitative Social Work*, 17(6), 849–864. https://doi.org/10.1177/1473250176994 5	To study social workers' occupational discussions on the complexities of their work in a Finnish social workers' trade union journal in 1958–1999.	Finnish social workers' accounts published in a professional trade paper in 1958–1999.	Archival study and identification of turning points in occupational culture.	Theories on professionalism, politization and critical theories of labour market transition.	The historical periodization of the occupational complexities indicates that social workers collectively reasserted the profession of social work and its institutional boundaries into a broader rubric of the demands brought about by changing society and the development of the Nordic welfare state.
Väänänen, A., Toivanen, M. and Lallukka, T. (2020). Lost in autonomy: Temporal structures and their implications for employees' autonomy and well-being among knowledge workers. *Occupational Health Science*, 4(1–2), 83–101. https://doi.org/10.1007/s41542-020-00058-1	To (1) explore and understand the temporal conditions framing work among autonomous knowledge professionals; (2) describe how autonomy is experienced in knowledge work jobs; and (3) analyse the implications of current autonomy for wellbeing in knowledge work.	Interviews of 21 women and 13 men who worked in knowledge-intensive jobs in Finland.	Thematic face-to-face interviews and content analysis.	Theories on stratification of time and time structures as well as critical reading of occupational health theories.	There are individual and social structures, and organizational and macro-level temporal structures in knowledge work. This creates a paradoxical nature of autonomy, characterized by high task autonomy and intense socio-temporal interdependence. Unsynchronized time structures can lead to fragmented work, overwhelming work burden, and higher risk of mental health problems.

(continued)

Table A.1: Original publications of the research group (continued)

Name	Aim	Material	Method	Theory	Main findings
Toivanen, M., Viljanen, O. and Turpeinen, M. (2016). Aikamatriiseja asiantuntijatyössä [Time matrices in expert work]. *Työelämän tutkimus [Work Life Research]*, 14(1), 77–94. https://journal.fi/tyoelamantutkimus/article/view/87024/45923	To recognize the temporal structures in which knowledge professionals work and to identify key characteristics characterizing knowledge-intensive work.	Interviews of 15 women and 11 men who worked in knowledge-intensive jobs.	Thematic face-to-face interviews and content analysis.	Theories on stratification of time and time structures in the context of late modern knowledge work.	Knowledge-intensive work is framed by both individual and social and organizational and macro-level time matrices. It is intertwined with the work of co-workers, the demands brought by email, the rhythm and habits of the organization and the pace and cycles of society.
Lehmuskoski, K., Väänänen, A., Juvonen-Posti, P. and Mattila-Holappa, P. (2022). Mielenterveyden toimijahahmot: Laadullinen tutkimus nuorista työntekijöistä kuntasektorilla [Social characters of mental health. A qualitative study of young employees in the municipal sector]. *Kuntoutus [Rehabilitation]*, 45(4), 6–19. https://doi.org/10.37451/kuntoutus.125397	To examine the work ability of young employees from the viewpoint of work life and cultural change. We also attempted to build a new kind of study-based viewpoint to support mental-health-related work ability.	70 interviews of young adults, occupational health service representatives, and supervisors from the municipal sector in the capital area of Finland in the year 2021.	Semi-structured interviews and content analysis.	Margaret Archer's theory of agency and the theory of social character.	Seven different social characters of young employee's mental health are presented in the results. The character typology shows that the mental health category has accumulated different challenges, which are intertwined with society, work and the individual life course, and are solved on an individual level by occupational health services. The diversity of a character's social and structural background highlights how mental vulnerability is structured as part of social and institutional action.

References

Abate, K.H., Abebe, Z., Abil, O.Z., Afshin, A., Ahmed, M.B., Alahdab, F. et al (2018). Global, regional, and national incidence, prevalence, and years lived with disability for 354 diseases and injuries for 195 countries and territories, 1990–2017: A systematic analysis for the Global Burden of Disease Study 2017. *The Lancet*, 392(10159), 1789–1858. https://doi.org/10.1016/S0140-6736(18)32279-7

Ackerknecht, E.H. (1967). A plea for a 'behaviorist' approach in writing the history of medicine. *Journal of the History of Medicine and Allied Sciences*, 22(3), 211–214.

Addis, M.E. and Mahalik, J.R. (2003). Men, masculinity, and the contexts of help seeking. *The American Psychologist*, 58(1), 5–14. https://doi.org/10.1037/0003-066x.58.1.5

Adkins, L. (1995). *Gendered Work: Sexuality, Family and the Labour Market*. Open University Press.

Ahtokari, R. (1992). *Vakuutusturvan puolesta: Suomen vakuutusyhtiöiden keskusliitto 1942–1992* [*Central Union of Insurances in Finland from 1942 to 1992*]. Suomen vakuutusyhtiöiden keskusliitto.

Alapuro, R. (2018). *State and Revolution in Finland*. Brill. https://brill.com/display/title/33518

Alasoini, T. (2012). Psykologinen sopimus organisaation ja työntekijöiden yhteisenä etuna [Psychological contract as a shared benefit of the organisation and employees]. In P. Pyöriä (ed), *Työhyvinvointi ja organisaation menestys* [*Occupational Well-Being and the Success of the Organisation*] (pp 99–108). Gaudeamus.

Alasuutari, P. (1996). *Toinen tasavalta: Suomi 1946–1994* [*Second Republic: Finland from 1946 to 1994*]. Vastapaino.

Alberti, G., Bessa, I., Hardy, K., Trappmann, V. and Umney, C. (2018). In, against and beyond precarity: Work in insecure times. *Work, Employment and Society*, 32(3), 447–457. https://doi.org/10.1177/0950017018762088

Albrecht, G.L. (2015). Bryan S. Turner: Bringing bodies and citizenship into the discussion of disability. In F. Collyer (ed), *The Palgrave Handbook of Social Theory in Health, Illness and Medicine* (pp 599–614). Palgrave Macmillan. https://doi.org/10.1057/9781137355621_38

Allen, B.J. (2004). *Difference Matters: Communicating Social Identity*. Waveland Press.

Alvesson, M. (2001). Knowledge work: Ambiguity, image and identity. *Human Relations*, 54(7), 863–886. https://doi.org/10.1177/0018726701547004

Amabile, T.M., Barsade, S.G., Mueller, J.S. and Staw, B.M. (2005). Affect and creativity at work. *Administrative Science Quarterly*, 50(3), 367–403. https://doi.org/10.2189/asqu.2005.50.3.367

Amable, B. (2003). *The Diversity of Modern Capitalism*. Oxford University Press.

American Psychiatric Association (2013). *Diagnostic and Statistical Manual of Mental Disorders: DSM-5™*. American Psychiatric Association.

Andersen, M.F., Svendsen, P.A., Nielsen, K., Brinkmann, S., Rugulies, R. and Madsen, I.E.H. (2022). Influence at work is a key factor for mental health: But what do contemporary employees in knowledge and relational work mean by 'influence at work'? *International Journal of Qualitative Studies on Health and Well-Being*, 17(1), 2054513. https://doi.org/10.1080/17482 631.2022.2054513

Anderson, B. (2010). Migration, immigration controls and the fashioning of precarious workers. *Work, Employment and Society*, 24(2), 300–317. https://doi.org/10.1177/0950017010362141

Andrews, F.M. and Withey, S.B. (1976). *Social Indicators of Well-Being: Americans' Perceptions of Life Quality*. Springer.

Annandale, E. and Clark, J. (2008). What is gender? Feminist theory and the sociology of human reproduction. *Sociology of Health & Illness*, 18, 17–44. https://doi.org/10.1111/1467-9566.ep10934409

Annandale, E., Harvey, J., Cavers, D. and Dixon-Woods, M. (2007). Gender and access to healthcare in the UK: A critical interpretive synthesis of the literature. *Evidence & Policy*, 3(4), 463–486. https://doi.org/10.1332/174 426407782516538

Anttila, E. and Väänänen, A. (2013). Rural schoolteachers and the pressures of community life: Local and cosmopolitan coping strategies in mid-twentieth-century Finland. *History of Education*, 42(2), 182–203. https://doi.org/10.1080/0046760X.2013.766267

Anttila, E. and Väänänen, A. (2015). From authority figure to emotion worker: Attitudes towards school discipline in Finnish schoolteachers' journals from the 1950s to the 1980s. *Pedagogy, Culture & Society*, 23(4), 555–574. https://doi.org/10.1080/14681366.2015.1015153

Anttila, E., Turtiainen, J., Varje, P. and Väänänen, A. (2018). Emotional labour in a school of individuals. *Pedagogy, Culture & Society*, 26(2), 215–231. https://doi.org/10.1080/14681366.2017.1378708

Archer, M.S. (2012). *The Reflexive Imperative in Late Modernity*. Cambridge University Press. https://doi.org/10.1017/CBO9781139108058

Arendt, H. (1998 [1958]). *The Human Condition*. University of Chicago Press.

Arikan, G. and Bloom, P. B.-N. (2015). Social values and cross-national differences in attitudes towards welfare. *Political Studies*, 63(2), 431–448. https://doi.org/10.1111/1467-9248.12100

Armstrong, D. (1995). The rise of surveillance medicine. *Sociology of Health & Illness*, 17(3), 393–404. https://doi.org/10.1111/1467-9566.ep10933329

Autor, D.H., Levy, F. and Murnane, R.J. (2003). The skill content of recent technological change: An empirical exploration. *The Quarterly Journal of Economics*, 118(4), 1279–1333. https://doi.org/10.1162/00335530332 2552801

Baines, D. and van den Broek, D. (2016). Coercive care: Control and coercion in the restructured care workplace. *British Journal of Social Work*, 47(1), 125–142. https://doi.org/10.1093/bjsw/bcw013

Baird, B., Smallwood, J., Mrazek, M., Kam, J., Franklin, M. and Schooler, J. (2012). Inspired by distraction: Mind wandering facilitates creative incubation. *Psychological Science*, 23(10), 1117–1122. https://doi.org/10.1177/0956797612446024

Bakhtin, M.M. (1981). *The Dialogic Imagination: Four Essays*. University of Texas Press.

Bakhtin, M.M. (1993). *Toward a Philosophy of the Act* (Vol 10). University of Texas Press.

Bakker, A.B. and Demerouti, E. (2007). The job demands-resources model: State of the art. *Journal of Managerial Psychology*, 22(3), 309–328. https://doi.org/10.1108/02683940710733115

Bakker, A.B. and Schaufeli, W.B. (2008). Positive organizational behavior: Engaged employees in flourishing organizations. *Journal of Organizational Behavior*, 29(2), 147–154. https://doi.org/10.1002/job.515

Barad, C. (1979). *Study of Burnout Syndrome Among Social Security Administration Field Public Contact Employees*. Social Security Administration.

Barley, S.R. and Kunda, G. (1992). Design and devotion: Surges of rational and normative ideologies of control in managerial discourse. *Administrative Science Quarterly*, 37(3), 363–399. https://doi.org/10.2307/2393449

Barling, J. and Griffiths, A. (2003). A history of occupational health psychology. In J.C. Quick and L.E. Tetrick (eds), *Handbook of Occupational Health Psychology* (pp 19–31). American Psychological Association. https://doi.org/10.1037/10474-002

Barnes, T. and Weller, S.A. (2020). Becoming precarious? Precarious work and life trajectories after retrenchment. *Critical Sociology*, 46(4–5), 527–541. https://doi.org/10.1177/0896920519896822

Bartholomew, T.T. and Brown, J.R. (2022). Entering the ethnographic mind: A grounded theory of using ethnography in psychological research. *Qualitative Research in Psychology*, 19(2), 316–345. https://doi.org/10.1080/14780887.2019.1604927

Baumeister, R.F. (1986). *Identity: Cultural Change and the Struggle for Self*. Oxford University Press.

Baumeister, R.F. and Muraven, M. (1996). Identity as adaptation to social, cultural, and historical context. *Journal of Adolescence*, 19(5), 405–416. https://doi.org/10.1006/jado.1996.0039

Baumeler, C. (2010). Organizational regimes of emotional conduct. In B. Sieben and Å. Wettergren (eds), *Emotionalizing Organizations and Organizing Emotions* (pp 272–292). Palgrave Macmillan.

Beard, G.M. (2008 [1881]). *American Nervousness, Its Causes and Consequences; a Supplement to Nervous Exhaustion (Neurasthenia) – Scholar's Choice Edition*. Putnam.

Beck, U. (1992). *Risk Society: Towards a New Modernity*. SAGE.

Beck, U. and Grande, E. (2010). Varieties of second modernity: The cosmopolitan turn in social and political theory and research. *The British Journal of Sociology*, 61(3), 409–443. https://doi.org/10.1111/j.1468-4446.2010.01320.x

Beehr, T.A. and Newman, J.E. (1978). Job stress, employee health, and organizational effectiveness: A facet analysis, model, and literature review. *Personnel Psychology*, 31(4), 665–699. https://doi.org/10.1111/j.1744-6570.1978.tb02118.x

Beeker, T., Mills, C., Bhugra, D., te Meerman, S., Thoma, S., Heinze, M. and von Peter, S. (2021). Psychiatrization of society: A conceptual framework and call for transdisciplinary research. *Frontiers in Psychiatry*, 12, 645556. https://doi.org/10.3389/fpsyt.2021.645556

Bell, D. (1973). *The Coming of Post-Industrial Society: A Venture in Social Forecasting*. Basic Books.

Bell, D. (1996). *The Cultural Contradictions of Capitalism. With a New Afterword by the Author*. Basic Books.

Benach, J., Vives, A., Tarafa, G., Delclos, C. and Muntaner, C. (2016). What should we know about precarious employment and health in 2025? Framing the agenda for the next decade of research. *International Journal of Epidemiology*, 45(1), 232–238. https://doi.org/10.1093/ije/dyv342

Bergholm, T. (2009). The making of the Finnish model: The qualitative change in Finnish corporatism in the early 1960s. *Scandinavian Journal of History*, 34(1), 29–48. https://doi.org/10.1080/03468750902770931

Bergholm, T. and Bieler, A. (2013). Globalization and the erosion of the Nordic model: A Swedish–Finnish comparison. *European Journal of Industrial Relations*, 19(1), 55–70. https://doi.org/10.1177/0959680112474747

Bericat, E. (2016). The sociology of emotions: Four decades of progress. *Current Sociology*, 64(3), 491–513. https://doi.org/10.1177/0011392115588355

Berlant, L.G. (2011). *Cruel Optimism*. Duke University Press.

Berlin, I. (1953). *The Hedgehog and the Fox: An Essay on Tolstoy's View of History*. Weidenfeld & Nicolson.

Berman, E., Bound, J. and Griliches, Z. (1994). Changes in the demand for skilled labor within U.S. manufacturing: Evidence from the annual survey of manufactures. *The Quarterly Journal of Economics*, 109(2), 367–397. https://doi.org/10.2307/2118467

Bhaskar, R. (1998). *The Possibility of Naturalism: A Philosophical Critique of the Contemporary Human Sciences*. Routledge. https://doi.org/10.4324/9780203976623

Bhatnagar, P., Wickramasinghe, K., Wilkins, E. and Townsend, N. (2016). Trends in the epidemiology of cardiovascular disease in the UK. *Heart*, 102(24), 1945–1952. https://doi.org/10.1136/heartjnl-2016-309573

Biehl, J., Good, B. and Kleinman, A. (2007). Introduction: Rethinking subjectivity. In J. Biehl, B. Good and A. Kleinman (eds), *Subjectivity: Ethnographic Investigations* (pp 1–23). University of California Press.

Blau, G. (1981). An empirical investigation of job stress, social support, service length, and job strain. *Organizational Behavior and Human Performance*, 27(2), 279–302. https://doi.org/10.1016/0030-5073(81)90050-7

Blaxter, M. (1976). Social class and health inequalities. In C.O. Carter and J. Peel (eds), *Equalities and Inequalities in Health* (pp 369–380). Academic Press.

Blayney, S. (2019). Industrial fatigue and the productive body: The science of work in Britain, c. 1900–1918. *Social History of Medicine: The Journal of the Society for the Social History of Medicine*, 32(2), 310–328. https://doi.org/10.1093/shm/hkx077

Blomgren, J. and Perhoniemi, R. (2022). Increase in sickness absence due to mental disorders in Finland: Trends by gender, age and diagnostic group in 2005–2019. *Scandinavian Journal of Public Health*, 50(3), 318–322. https://doi.org/10.1177/1403494821993705

Bohan, J.S. (1993). Regarding gender: Essentialism, constructionism, and feminist psychology. *Psychology of Women Quarterly*, 17(1), 5–21. https://doi.org/10.1111/j.1471-6402.1993.tb00673.x

Boltanski, L. and Chiapello, E. (2007). *The New Spirit of Capitalism*. Verso Books.

Bolton, S. (2005). *Emotion Management in the Workplace*. Palgrave Macmillan.

Bolton, S. and Boyd, C. (2003). Trolley dolly or skilled emotion manager? Moving on from Hochschild's managed heart. *Work, Employment and Society*, 17(2), 289–308. https://doi.org/10.1177/0950017003017002004

Bosmans, K., Hardonk, S., De Cuyper, N. and Vanroelen, C. (2016). Explaining the relation between precarious employment and mental well-being: A qualitative study among temporary agency workers. *Work*, 53(2), 249–264. https://doi.org/10.3233/WOR.152136

Bosqui, T., Väänänen, A., Buscariolli, A., Koskinen, A., O'Reilly, D., Airila, A. and Kouvonen, A. (2019). Antidepressant medication use among working age first-generation migrants resident in Finland: An administrative data linkage study. *International Journal for Equity in Health*, 18(1), 157. https://doi.org/10.1186/s12939-019-1060-9

Bosqui, T., Väänänen, A., Koskinen, A., Buscariolli, A., O'Reilly, D., Airila, A., Toivanen, M. and Kouvonen, A. (2020). Antipsychotic medication use among working-age first-generation migrants resident in Finland: An administrative data linkage study. *Scandinavian Journal of Public Health*, 48(1), 64–71. https://doi.org/10.1177/1403494819841960

Bourdieu, P. (1984). *Distinction: A Social Critique of the Judgement of Taste*. Harvard University Press.

Bovet, P. (2014). *Epidemiologic Transition, Global Burden of Disease, and Emergence of NCDs*. 8th WHO-IUMSP International Seminar on the Public Health Aspects of NCDs, Lausanne-Geneva. http://doczz.net/doc/7977769/health-transition-gbd-bovet-

Boxall, P. and Macky, K. (2014). High-involvement work processes, work intensification and employee well-being. *Work, Employment and Society*, 28(6), 963–984. https://doi.org/10.1177/0950017013512714

Boysen, G., Ebersole, A., Casner, R. and Coston, N. (2014). Gendered mental disorders: Masculine and feminine stereotypes about mental disorders and their relation to stigma. *The Journal of Social Psychology*, 154(6), 546–565. https://doi.org/10.1080/00224545.2014.953028

Braidotti, R. (2019). *Posthuman Knowledge*. Polity Press.

Braverman, H. (1974). *Labor and Monopoly Capital: The Degradation of Work in the Twentieth Century*. Monthly Review Press.

Brinkmann, S. (2016). *Diagnostic Cultures: A Cultural Approach to the Pathologization of Modern Life*. Routledge.

Bröer, C. and Besseling, B. (2017). Sadness or depression: Making sense of low mood and the medicalization of everyday life. *Social Science & Medicine*, 183, 28–36. https://doi.org/10.1016/j.socscimed.2017.04.025

Broom, A. (2005). Medical specialists' accounts of the impact of the internet on the doctor/patient relationship. *Health*, 9(3), 319–338. https://doi.org/10.1177/1363459305052903

Broom, D.H. and Woodward, R.V. (1996). Medicalisation reconsidered: Toward a collaborative approach to care. *Sociology of Health & Illness*, 18(3), 357–378. https://doi.org/10.1111/1467-9566.ep10934730

Brown, P., Elston, M.A. and Gabe, J. (2015). From patient deference towards negotiated and precarious informality: An Eliasian analysis of English general practitioners' understandings of changing patient relations. *Social Science & Medicine*, 146, 164–172. https://doi.org/10.1016/j.socscimed.2015.10.047

Brownlie, J. (2011). Not 'going there': Limits to the professionalisation of our emotional lives. *Sociology of Health & Illness*, 33(1), 130–144. https://doi.org/10.1111/j.1467-9566.2010.01269.x

Brun, E. and Milczarek, M. (2007). *Expert Forecast on Emerging Psychosocial Risks Related to Occupational Safety and Health* (5; European Risk Observatory Report). European Agency for Safety and Health at Work.

Brunila, K. (2012). A diminished self: Entrepreneurial and therapeutic ethos operating with a common aim. *European Educational Research Journal*, 11(4), 477–486. https://doi.org/10.2304/eerj.2012.11.4.477

Burawoy, M. (1979). *Manufacturing Consent: Changes in the Labor Process Under Monopoly Capitalism*. University of Chicago Press.

Burawoy, M. (2012). The roots of domination: Beyond Bourdieu and Gramsci. *Sociology*, 46(2), 187–206. https://doi.org/10.1177/0038038511422725

Buscariolli, A., Kouvonen, A., Kokkinen, L., Halonen, J.I., Koskinen, A. and Väänänen, A. (2018). Human service work, gender and antidepressant use: A nationwide register-based 19-year follow-up of 752 683 women and men. *Occupational and Environmental Medicine*, 75(6), 401–406. https://doi.org/10.1136/oemed-2017-104803

Busfield, J. (2000). Introduction: Rethinking the sociology of mental health. *Sociology of Health & Illness*, 22(5), 543–558. https://doi.org/10.1111/1467-9566.00219

Busfield, J. (2011). *Mental Illness*. Polity Press.

Busse, C., Mahlendorf, M.D. and Bode, C. (2016). The ABC for studying the too-much-of-a-good-thing effect: A competitive mediation framework linking antecedents, benefits, and costs. *Organizational Research Methods*, 19(1), 131–153. https://doi.org/10.1177/1094428115579699

Butler, J. (2006 [1990]). *Gender Trouble: Feminism and the Subversion of Identity*. Routledge.

Cabanas, E. and Illouz, E. (2019). *Manufacturing Happy Citizens: How the Science and Industry of Happiness Control Our Lives*. Polity Press.

Campbell, I. and Price, R. (2016). Precarious work and precarious workers: Towards an improved conceptualisation. *The Economic and Labour Relations Review*, 27(3), 314–332. https://doi.org/10.1177/1035304616652074

Cannon, W.B. (1932). *The Wisdom of the Body*. W.W. Norton.

Carey, M. (2007). White-collar proletariat? Braverman, the deskilling/upskilling of social work and the paradoxical life of the agency care manager. *Journal of Social Work*, 7(1), 93–114. https://doi.org/10.1177/1468017307075992

Carlgren, I., Klette, K., Mýrdal, S., Schnack, K. and Simola, H. (2006). Changes in Nordic teaching practices: From individualised teaching to the teaching of individuals. *Scandinavian Journal of Educational Research*, 50(3), 301–326. https://doi.org/10.1080/00313830600743357

Cascio, W.F. (1995). Whither industrial and organizational psychology in a changing world of work? *The American Psychologist*, 50(11), 928–939. https://doi.org/10.1037/0003-066X.50.11.928

Castells, M. (1996). The net and the self: Working notes for a critical theory of the informational society. *Critique of Anthropology*, 16(1), 9–38. https://doi.org/10.1177/0308275X9601600103

Castelpietra, G., Knudsen, A.K.S., Agardh, E.E., Armocida, B., Beghi, M., Iburg, K.M. et al (2022). The burden of mental disorders, substance use disorders and self-harm among young people in Europe, 1990–2019: Findings from the Global Burden of Disease Study 2019. *The Lancet Regional Health – Europe*, 16, 100341. https://doi.org/10.1016/j.lanepe.2022.100341

Cederström, C. and Spicer, A. (2015). *The Wellness Syndrome*. Polity Press.

Chaplin, T.M. (2015). Gender and emotion expression: A developmental contextual perspective. *Emotion Review*, 7(1), 14–21. https://doi.org/10.1177/1754073914544408

Charles, C., Gafni, A. and Whelan, T. (1999). Decision-making in the physician–patient encounter: Revisiting the shared treatment decision-making model. *Social Science & Medicine*, 49(5), 651–661. https://doi.org/10.1016/s0277-9536(99)00145-8

Charlesworth, S.J. (2000). *A Phenomenology of Working Class Experience*. Cambridge University Press.

Chesley, N. (2014). Information and communication technology use, work intensification and employee strain and distress. *Work, Employment and Society*, 28(4), 589–610. https://doi.org/10.1177/0950017013500112

Choi, B. (2020). Developing a job exposure matrix of work organization hazards in the United States: A review on methodological issues and research protocol. *Safety and Health at Work*, 11(4), 397–404. https://doi.org/10.1016/j.shaw.2020.05.007

Choi, B.K., Schnall, P., Landsbergis, P., Dobson, M., Ko, S., Gómez-Ortiz, V., Juárez-Garcia, A. and Baker, D. (2015). Recommendations for individual participant data meta-analyses on work stressors and health outcomes: Comments on IPD-work consortium papers. *Scandinavian Journal of Work, Environment & Health*, 41(3), 299–311. https://doi.org/10.5271/sjweh.3484

Clausen, C. and Olsen, P. (2000). Strategic management and the politics of production in the development of work: A case study in a Danish electronic manufacturing plant. *Technology Analysis & Strategic Management*, 12(1), 59–74. https://doi.org/10.1080/095373200107238

Clement, W., Mathieu, S., Prus, S. and Uckardesler, E. (2009). Precarious lives in the new economy: Comparative intersectional analysis. In L.F. Vosko, M. MacDonald and I. Campbell (eds), *Gender and the Contours of Precarious Employment*. Routledge.

Collier, S.J. (2011). *Post-Soviet Social: Neoliberalism, Social Modernity, Biopolitics*. Princeton University Press.

Collingwood, R.G. (1946). *The Idea of History*. Edited by T.M. Knox. Oxford University Press.

Collinson, D.L. (2010). *Managing the Shopfloor: Subjectivity, Masculinity and Workplace Culture*. Walter de Gruyter.

Connell, R.W. (1995). *Masculinities*. University of California Press.

Connelly, J. and Costall, A. (2000). R.G. Collingwood and the idea of a historical psychology. *Theory & Psychology*, 10(2), 147–170. https://doi.org/10.1177/0959354300102001

Conrad, P. (2007). *The Medicalization of Society: On the Transformation of Human Conditions into Treatable Disorders*. Johns Hopkins University Press.

Cooper, C. and Dewe, P.J. (2008). *Stress: A Brief History*. John Wiley & Sons.

Cooper, C., Goswami, U. and Sahakian, B.J. (2010). *Mental Capital and Wellbeing*. Wiley-Blackwell.

Cooper, C.L. and Marshall, J. (1978). *Understanding Executive Stress*. Macmillan.

Côté, J.E. (2019). *Youth Development in Identity Societies: Paradoxes of Purpose*. Routledge.

Cottingham, M.D. (2016). Theorizing emotional capital. *Theory and Society*, 45(5), 451–470. https://doi.org/10.1007/s11186-016-9278-7

Courtenay, W.H. (2000). Constructions of masculinity and their influence on men's well-being: A theory of gender and health. *Social Science & Medicine*, 50(10), 1385–1401. https://doi.org/10.1016/S0277-9536(99)00390-1

Crawford, R. (1994). The boundaries of the self and the unhealthy other: Reflections on health, culture and AIDS. *Social Science & Medicine*, 38(10), 1347–1365. https://doi.org/10.1016/0277-9536(94)90273-9

Crutzen, P. (2000). The 'anthropocene'. *The International Geosphere–Biosphere Programme (IGBP): Global Change Newsletter*, 41, 17–18.

Danziger, K. (1997). *Naming the Mind: How Psychology Found Its Language*. SAGE.

Demirkan, A., Penninx, B., Hek, K., Wray, N.R., Amin, N., Aulchenko, Y.S. et al (2011). Genetic risk profiles for depression and anxiety in adult and elderly cohorts. *Molecular Psychiatry*, 16(7), 773–783. https://doi.org/10.1038/mp.2010.65

De Vos, J. (2013). *Psychologization and the Subject of Late Modernity*. Springer.

Dew, M.A., Bromet, E.J., Schulberg, H.C., Parkinson, D.K. and Curtis, E.C. (1991). Factors affecting service utilization for depression in a white collar population. *Social Psychiatry and Psychiatric Epidemiology*, 26(5), 230–237. https://doi.org/10.1007/BF00788971

de Wolff, C.J. (1994). Human resources management in Western organizations. *European Work and Organizational Psychologist*, 4(3). https://doi.org/10.1080/13594329408410485

Diener, E., Suh, E.M., Lucas, R.E. and Smith, H.L. (1999). Subjective well-being: Three decades of progress. *Psychological Bulletin*, 125(2), 276–302. https://doi.org/10.1037/0033-2909.125.2.276

Dixon, T. (2012). 'Emotion': The history of a keyword in crisis. *Emotion Review*, 4(4), 338–344. https://doi.org/10.1177/1754073912445814

Doblhofer, D.S., Hauser, A., Kuonath, A., Haas, K., Agthe, M. and Frey, D. (2019). Make the best out of the bad: Coping with value incongruence through displaying facades of conformity, positive reframing, and self-disclosure. *European Journal of Work and Organizational Psychology*, 28(5), 572–593. https://doi.org/10.1080/1359432X.2019.1567579

Doblytė, S. (2019). Bourdieu's theory of fields: Towards understanding help-seeking practices in mental distress. *Social Theory & Health*, 17(3), 273–290. https://doi.org/10.1057/s41285-019-00105-0

Dolan, A. (2011). 'You can't ask for a Dubonnet and lemonade!': Working class masculinity and men's health practices. *Sociology of Health & Illness*, 33(4), 586–601. https://doi.org/10.1111/j.1467-9566.2010.01300.x

Dragus, J.G. (1996). Abnormal behaviour in Chinese societies: Clinical, epidemiological, and comparative studies. In M. Harris (ed), *The Oxford Handbook of Chinese Psychology* (pp 412–428). Oxford University Press.

Dunne, J. (1995). Beyond sovereignty and deconstruction: The storied self. *Philosophy & Social Criticism*, 21(5–6), 137–157. https://doi.org/10.1177/0191453795021005-611

Durkheim, É. (1964). *The Rules of Sociological Method* (8th edn). The Free Press.

Durkheim, É. (1965). *The Elementary Forms of the Religious Life*. The Free Press.

Eakin, J. (1997). Work-related determinants of health behavior. In D.S. Gochman (ed), *Handbook of Health Behavior Research I: Personal and Social Determinants* (pp 337–357). Plenum Press.

Eaton, W., Muntaner, C. and Sapag, J.C. (2010). Socioeconomic stratification and mental disorder. In T.L. Scheid and T.N. Brown (eds), *A Handbook for the Study of Mental Health: Social Contexts, Theories, and Systems* (pp 226–255). Cambridge University Press.

Ecclestone, K. and Hayes, D. (2009). *The Dangerous Rise of Therapeutic Education*. Routledge.

Eggenberger, L., Fordschmid, C., Ludwig, C., Weber, S., Grub, J., Komlenac, N. and Walther, A. (2021). Men's psychotherapy use, male role norms, and male-typical depression symptoms: Examining 716 men and women experiencing psychological distress. *Behavioral Sciences*, 11(6), 83.

Ehrenberg, A. (1991). *Le Culte de la Performance*. Calmann-Lévy.

Ehrenberg, A. (2010). *Weariness of the Self: Diagnosing the History of Depression in the Contemporary Age*. McGill-Queen's Press.

Ehrenberg, A. (2017). What we talk about when we talk about mental health: Towards an anthropology of adversity in individualistic society. In S. Neckel, A.K. Schaffner and G. Wagner (eds), *Burnout, Fatigue, Exhaustion: An Interdisciplinary Perspective on a Modern Affliction* (pp 153–171). Springer.

Ehrenreich, B. (1989). *Fear of Falling: The Inner Life of the Middle Class*. Pantheon Books.

Ehrenreich, B. (2019). *Natural Causes: An Epidemic of Wellness, the Certainty of Dying, and Killing Ourselves to Live Longer*. Twelve.

Elias, N. (1978). *What is Sociology?* Columbia University Press.

Elias, N. (1991). *The Society of Individuals*. Blackwell.

Elias, N. (1994). *Civilizing Process*. Blackwell.

Elston, M.A. (2009). Remaking a trustworthy profession in twenty-first century Britain. In J. Gabe and M. Calnan (eds), *The New Sociology of Health Service* (pp 17–36). Routledge.

Emery, F.E. and Thorsrud, E. (eds) (2013 [1969]). *Form and Content in Industrial Democracy: Some Experiences from Norway and Other European Countries*. Routledge. https://doi.org/10.4324/9781315013695

Encyclopedia of Population (2019). *Health Transition*. Encyclopedia.Com. https://www.encyclopedia.com/social-sciences/encyclopedias-almanacs-transcripts-and-maps/health-transition

Engels, F. (2001 [1845]). *The Condition of the Working Class in England*. Electric Book Co.

Ericson, R.J. and Stacey, C.L. (2013). Attending to mind and body: Engaging the complexity of emotion practice among caring professionals. In A. Grandey, J.M. Diefendorff and D.E. Rupp (eds), *Emotional Labor in the 21st Century: Diverse Perspectives on the Psychology of Emotion Regulation at Work* (pp 175–196). Routledge Academic.

Eriksen, T.H. (2016). *Overheating: An Anthropology of Accelerated Change*. Pluto Press.

Erikson, E.H. (1963). *Childhood and Society*. W.W. Norton & Company.

Ervasti, J., Kausto, J., Leino-Arjas, P., Turunen, J., Varje, P. and Väänänen, A. (2022). *Työkyvyn tuen vaikuttavuus Tutkimuskatsaus työkyvyn tukitoimien työkyky- ja kustannusvaikutuksista* [*Effectiveness of Interventions to Support Work Ability and Prevent Work Disability. Review on Effects and Cost Effectiveness*] [Sarjajulkaisu], 26 January. Valtioneuvoston kanslia [Prime Minister's Office]. https://julkaisut.valtioneuvosto.fi/handle/10024/163779

Eurostat (2022). *Precarious Employment by Sex, Age and NACE*. https://app sso.eurostat.ec.europa.eu/nui/show.do?dataset=lfsa_qoe_4ax1r2&lang=en

Ezzy, D. (2001). A simulacrum of workplace community: Individualism and engineered culture. *Sociology*, 35(3), 631–650. https://doi.org/10.1017/S0038038501000323

Fawcett, B. (2009). Vulnerability: Questioning the certainties in social work and health. *International Social Work*, 52(4), 473–484. https://doi.org/10.1177/0020872809104251

Fejes, A. and Dahlstedt, M. (2013). *The Confessing Society: Foucault, Confession and Practices of Lifelong Learning*. Routledge

Fellman, S. (2008). Growth and investment: Finnish capitalism, 1850–2005. In S. Fellman, M.J. Iversen, H. Sjögren and L. Thue (eds), *Creating Nordic Capitalism: The Business History of a Competitive Periphery* (pp 139–217). Palgrave Macmillan.

Ferrari, A.J., Santomauro, D.F., Herrera, A.M.M., Shadid, J., Ashbaugh, C., Erskine, H.E. et al (2022). Global, regional, and national burden of 12 mental disorders in 204 countries and territories, 1990–2019: A systematic analysis for the Global Burden of Disease Study 2019. *The Lancet. Psychiatry*, 9(2), 137–150. https://doi.org/10.1016/S2215-0366(21)00395-3

Ferrie, J.E., Virtanen, M. and Kivimaki, M. (2014). The healthy population–high disability paradox. *Occupational and Environmental Medicine*, 71(4), 232–233. https://doi.org/10.1136/oemed-2013-101945

Figert, A.E. (1996). *Women and the Ownership of PMS: The Structuring of a Psychiatric Disorder*. Aldine Transaction.

Fineman, S. (2010). Emotion in organizations – a critical turn. In B. Sieben and Å. Wettergren (eds), *Emotionalizing Organizations and Organizing Emotions* (pp 23–41). Palgrave Macmillan.

Finnish Centre for Pensions (2022). *Statistical Database*. https://tilastot.etk.fi/pxweb/en/ETK

Fleming, P.J. and Agnew-Brune, C. (2015). Current trends in the study of gender norms and health behaviors. *Current Opinion in Psychology*, 5, 72–77. https://doi.org/10.1016/j.copsyc.2015.05.001

Flick, U. (2018). Doing triangulation and mixed methods. *Doing Triangulation and Mixed Methods*. https://doi.org/10.4135/9781529716634

Forma, P. (2023). *Johtajan työkykykirja* [*A Book on Work Ability for Leaders*]. Alma Talent Bisneskirjasto.

Foucault, M. (1973). *The Birth of the Clinic: An Archaeology of Medical Perception*. Routledge.

Foucault, M. (1984). On the genealogy of ethics: An overview of work in progress. In *The Foucault Reader* (pp 340–372). Pantheon Books.

Foucault, M. (1988). The ethic of the care for the self as a practice of freedom: An interview with Michael Foucault on 20th January 1984. In J. Bernauer and D.M. Rasmussen (eds), *The Final Foucault* (pp 1–20). MIT Press.

Foucault, M. (2003). *Madness and Civilization*. Routledge.

Foucault, M. (2005). *The Order of Things: An Archaeology of the Human Sciences*. Routledge.

Fowers, B.J., Novak, L.F., Calder, A.J. and Sommer, R.K. (2021). The distorting lens of psychology's individualism and a social realist alternative. In B.D. Slife, S.C. Yanchar and F.C. Richardson (eds), *Routledge International Handbook of Theoretical and Philosophical Psychology* (pp 78–97). Routledge.

Frankenhaeuser, M. and Gardell, B. (1976). Underload and overload in working life: Outline of a multidisciplinary approach. *Journal of Human Stress*, 2(3), 35–46. https://doi.org/10.1080/0097840X.1976.9936068

Freudenberger, H.J. (1974). Staff burn-out. *Journal of Social Issues*, 30(1), 159–165. https://doi.org/10.1111/j.1540-4560.1974.tb00706.x

Friberg, T. (2009). Burnout: From popular culture to psychiatric diagnosis in Sweden. *Culture, Medicine and Psychiatry*, 33(4), 538–558. https://doi.org/10.1007/s11013-009-9149-z

Frommer, J. and Frommer, S. (1993). Max Weber's illness: Sociologic aspects of the depressive structure. *Fortschritte Der Neurologie-Psychiatrie* [*Advances in Neurology-Psychiatry*], 61(5), 161–171. https://doi.org/10.1055/s-2007-999084

Frommer, J. and Frommer, S. (1998). Max Weber's disease: Research on the disease and therapeutic management at the turn of the century. *Fortschritte Der Neurologie-Psychiatrie [Advances in Neurology-Psychiatry]*, 66(5), 193–200. https://doi.org/10.1055/s-2007-995255

Furedi, F. (2004). *Therapy Culture: Cultivating Vulnerability in an Uncertain Age*. Routledge.

Furusten, S. (2003). *God managementkonsultation: Reglerad expertis eller improviserat artisteri? [Good Management Consulting: Regulated Expertise or Improvised Artistery?]*. Studentlitteratur [Student Literature].

Fusco, C. (2006). Inscribing healthification: Governance, risk, surveillance and the subjects and spaces of fitness and health. *Health & Place*, 12(1), 65–78. https://doi.org/10.1016/j.healthplace.2004.10.003

Gabe, J. and Bury, M. (1988). Tranquillizers as a social problem. *Sociological Review*, 36(2), 320–352.

Gallie, D. (ed). (2007). *Employment Regimes and the Quality of Work*. Oxford University Press. https://doi.org/10.1093/acprof:oso/9780199230 105.001.0001

Gardell, B. (1976). *Arbetsinnehåll och livskvalitet: En sammanställning och diskussion av samhällsvetenskaplig forskning rörande människan och arbetet [The Content of Work and the Guality of Life]*. Prisma.

Garsten, C. (2008). *Workplace Vagabonds: Career and Community in Changing Worlds of Work*. Springer.

Geertz, C. (1973). Deep play: Notes on the Balinese cockfight. In C. Geertz, *The Interpretation of Cultures: Selected Essays* (pp 412–453). Basic Books.

Geertz, C. (1983). Local knowledge: Fact and law in comparative perspective. In *Local Knowledge: Further Essays in Interpretive Anthropology* (pp 167–234). Basic Books.

Gergen, K.J. (1973). Social psychology as history. *Journal of Personality and Social Psychology*, 26(2), 309–320. https://doi.org/10.1037/h0034436

Gergen, K.J. (1991). *The Saturated Self: Dilemmas of Identity in Contemporary Life*. Basic Books.

Gerth, H. and Mills, C.W. (1954). *Character and Social Structure: The Psychology of Social Institutions*. Routledge & Kegan.

Giddens, A. (1984). *The Constitution of Society: Outline of the Theory of Structuration*. Polity.

Giddens, A. (1991). *Modernity and Self-Identity: Self and Society in the Late Modern Age*. Stanford University Press.

Goffman, E. (1961). *Asylums: Essays on the Social Situation of Mental Patients and Other Inmates*. Aldine.

Golder, B. (2007). Foucault and the genealogy of pastoral power. *Radical Philosophy Review*, 10(2), 157–176.

Goleman, D. (1996). *Emotional Intelligence: Why It Can Matter More Than IQ*. Bloomsbury.

Gorz, A. (1999). *Reclaiming Work: Beyond the Wage-Based Society*. Polity.

Green, F. (2004). Why has work effort become more intense? *Industrial Relations*, 43(4), 709–741. https://doi.org/10.1111/j.0019-8676.2004.00359.x

Green, F. (2006). *Demanding Work: The Paradox of Job Quality in the Affluent Economy*. Princeton University Press.

Greenfeld, L. (1992). *Nationalism: Five Roads to Modernity*. Harvard University Press.

Grob, G.N. (1991). Origins of DSM-I: A study in appearance and reality. *The American Journal of Psychiatry*, 148(4), 421–431. https://doi.org/10.1176/ajp.148.4.421

Grzywacz, J.G., Butler, A.B. and Almeida, D.M. (2008). Work, family, and health: Work–family balance as a protective factor against stresses of daily life. In A. Marcus-Newhall, D.F. Halpern and S.J. Tan (eds), *The Changing Realities of Work and Family* (pp 194–215). John Wiley & Sons. https://doi.org/10.1002/9781444305272.ch10

Guignon, C. (1990). Truth as disclosure: Art, language, history. *The Southern Journal of Philosophy*, 28(S1), 105–120. https://doi.org/10.1111/j.2041-6962.1990.tb00569.x

Guillén, M.F. (1994). *Models of Management: Work, Authority and Organization in a Comparative Perspective*. University of Chicago Press.

Haapala, P. (2004). Väki vähenee–maatalousyhteiskunnan hidas häviö 1950–2000 [The slow defeat of the agrarian society 1950–2000]. In P. Markkola (eds), *Suomen Maatalouden Historia III. Suurten Muutosten Aika. Jälleenrakennuskaudesta EU-Suomeen* [*The History of Finland's Agriculture III. The Time of Great Changes. From the Era of Rebuilding to the EU Finland*]. *Suomalaisen Kirjallisuuden Seuran Toimituksia* [*The Editions of Finnish Literature Society*], 914(3), 233–254.

Haapala, P. (2006). Suomalainen rakennemuutos [Restructuring in Finland]. In J. Saari (ed), *Historiallinen käänne. Johdatus pitkän aikavälin historian tutkimukseen* [*Historical Turn: Introduction in Long-Term Historical Research*] (pp 91–124). Gaudeamus.

Hacking, I. (1995). The looping effects of human kinds. In D. Sperber, D. Premack and A. Premack (eds), *Causal Cognition: A Multidisciplinary Debate* (pp 351–349). Clarendon Press.

Hacking, I. (1999). *The Social Construction of What?* Harvard University Press.

Hackman, J.R. and Oldham, G.R. (1976). Motivation through the design of work: Test of a theory. *Organizational Behavior and Human Performance*, 16(2), 250–279. https://doi.org/10.1016/0030-5073(76)90016-7

Hakala, K., Björnsdóttir, K., Lappalainen, S., Jóhannesson, I.Á. and Teittinen, A. (2018). Nordic perspectives on disability studies in education: A review of research in Finland and Iceland. *Education Inquiry*, 9(1), 78–96. https://doi.org/10.1080/20004508.2017.1421390

Häkkinen, A. and Salasuo, M. (2016). Sukupolvet ja hyvä elämä [Generations and good life]. In S. Myllyniemi (ed), *Arjen jäljillä Nuorisobarometri 2015* [*The Youth Barometer 2015*] (pp 183–192). Nuorisotutkimusverkosto.

Hakulinen, C., Elovainio, M., Arffman, M., Lumme, S., Pirkola, S., Keskimäki, I., Manderbacka, K. and Böckerman, P. (2019). Mental disorders and long-term labour market outcomes: Nationwide cohort study of 2 055 720 individuals. *Acta Psychiatrica Scandinavica*, 140(4), 371–381. https://doi.org/10.1111/acps.13067

Hakulinen, C., Komulainen, K., Suokas, K., Pirkola, S., Pulkki-Råback, L., Lumme, S., Elovainio, M. and Böckerman, P. (2023). Socioeconomic position at the age of 30 and the later risk of a mental disorder: A nationwide population-based register study. *Journal of Epidemiology and Community Health*, 77(5), 298–304. https://doi.org/10.1136/jech-2022-219674

Halfmann, D. (2012). Recognizing medicalization and demedicalization: Discourses, practices, and identities. *Health*, 16(2), 186–207. https://doi.org/10.1177/1363459311403947

Hall, P.A. and Soskice, D. (2001). An introduction to *Varieties of Capitalism*. In P.A. Hall and D. Soskice (eds), *Varieties of Capitalism: The Institutional Foundations of Comparative Advantage* (pp 1–68). Oxford University Press.

Halonen, J.I., Koskinen, A., Varje, P., Kouvonen, A., Hakanen, J.J. and Väänänen, A. (2018a). Mental health by gender-specific occupational groups: Profiles, risks and dominance of predictors. *Journal of Affective Disorders*, 238, 311–316. https://doi.org/10.1016/j.jad.2018.06.007

Halonen, J.I., Koskinen, A., Kouvonen, A., Varje, P., Pirkola, S. and Väänänen, A. (2018b). Distinctive use of newer and older antidepressants in major geographical areas: A nationally representative register-based study. *Journal of Affective Disorders*, 229, 358–363. https://doi.org/10.1016/j.jad.2017.12.102

Hämäläinen, P., Saarela, K.L. and Takala, J. (2009). Global trend according to estimated number of occupational accidents and fatal work-related diseases at region and country level. *Journal of Safety Research*, 40(2), 125–139. https://doi.org/10.1016/j.jsr.2008.12.010

Hammersley, M. and Atkinson, P. (2019). *Ethnography: Principles in Practice* (4th edn). Routledge.

Hannikainen, M. and Heikkinen, S. (2006). The labour market, 1850–2000. In J. Ojala, J. Eloranta and J. Jalava (eds), *The Road to Prosperity: An Economic History of Finland* (pp 165–186). SKS.

Hänninen, V. (1987). *Työ, elämäntapa, psyykkinen hyvinvointi* [*Work, Lifestyle, Mental Well-Being*]. Tampereen yliopisto [University of Tampere].

Hargreaves, A. (1998). The emotional practice of teaching. *Teaching and Teacher Education*, 14(8), 835–854. https://doi.org/10.1016/S0742-051X(98)00025-0

Harkness, A.M.B., Long, B.C., Bermbach, N., Patterson, K., Jordan, S. and Kahn, H. (2005). Talking about work stress. Discourse analysis and implications for stress interventions. *Work and Stress*, 19(2), 121–136. https://doi.org/10.1080/02678370500160068

Harvey, D. (2005). *A Brief History of Neoliberalism*. Oxford University Press.

Haslam, N. (2005). Dimensions of folk psychiatry. *Review of General Psychology*, 9(1), 35–47. https://doi.org/10.1037/1089-2680.9.1.35

Häusser, J.A., Mojzisch, A., Niesel, M, and Schulz-Hardt, S. (2010). Ten years on: A review of recent research on the Job Demand–Control (-Support) model and psychological well-being. *Work & Stress*, 24(1), 1–35. https://doi.org/10.1080/02678371003683747

Health and Safety Executive (2019). *Work-related Stress, Depression or Anxiety Statistics in Great Britain 2019*. Health and Safety Executive. hse.gov.uk.

Heidegger, M. (1962). *Being and Time*. Harper.

Heiskala, R. (1994). Silmänkääntäjä, jutunkertoja ja vuorovaikutuksen tutkija. Ensimmäinen kokonaisesitys sosiologi Erving Goffmanista [Erving Goffman: Conjurer, storyteller and researcher of interaction]. *Helsingin Sanomat*, 19 December.

Helén, I. (2007a). Masennuksen historiat [Histories of depression]. *Psykologia [Psychology]*, 42(3), 196–210, 243.

Helén, I. (2007b). Masennus massamitassa: Epidemiologinen välineistö ja psykiatrian muodonmuutos [Extensive depression: Epidemiologic tools and the transformation of psychiatry]. *Tiede & Edistys [Science & Progress]*, 32(2). https://doi.org/10.51809/te.104883

Helén, I. (2010). Psykiatrian muodonmuutos ja depression nousu kansantaudiksi. Historiallis-sosiologinen interventio [Transformation of psychiatry and rise of depression as endemic disease: Historical and sociological intervention]. *Sosiaalilääketieteellinen Aikakauslehti [Finnish Social Medicine Journal]*, 47(1).

Hellgren, J., Sverke, M. and Näswall, K. (2008a). Changing work roles: New demands and challenges. In K. Naswall, J. Hellgren and M. Sverke (eds), *The Individual in the Changing Working Life* (pp 46–66). Cambridge University Press. https://doi.org/10.1017/CBO9780511490064

Hellgren, J., Sverke, M. and Näswall, K. (2008b). The individual in the changing working life: Introduction. In K. Naswall, J. Hellgren and M. Sverke (eds), *The Individual in the Changing Working Life* (pp 1–16). Cambridge University Press. https://doi.org/10.1017/CBO9780511 1490064

Hemmings, P. and Prinz, C. (2020). Sickness and disability systems: Comparing outcomes and policies in Norway with those in Sweden, the Netherlands and Switzerland. *OECD Economics Department Working Papers*, No. 1601, OECD Publishing. https://doi.org/10.1787/c768699b-en

Herring, J. (2016). *Vulnerable Adults and the Law*. Oxford University Press. https://doi.org/10.1093/acprof:oso/9780198737278.001.0001

Herzberg, F. (1968). *One More Time: How Do You Motivate Employees* (Vol 65). Harvard Business Review. http://mcrhrdi.gov.in/91fc/coursemater ial/management/14%20One%20More%20Time%20How%20do%20 you%20Motivate%20Employees.pdf

Hillert, A., Sandman, J., Ehmig, S.C., Weisbecker, H., Kepplinger, H.M. and Benkert, O. (1999). The general public's cognitive and emotional perception of mental illnesses: An alternative to attitude-research. In J. Guimón and W. Fischer (eds), *The Image of Madness: The Public Facing Mental Illness and Psychiatric Treatment* (pp 56–71). Karger Medical and Scientific Publishers.

Hillson, D. and Murray-Webster, R. (2005). *Understanding and Managing Risk Attitude*. Gower Publishing.

Hillson, D. and Murray-Webster, R. (2006). *Managing Risk Attitude Using Emotional Literacy*. PMI® Global Congress 2006 – EMEA, Newtown Square, PA. https://www.pmi.org/learning/library/managing-risk-attit ude-using-emotional-literacy-8156

Hochschild, A.R. (1979). Emotion work, feeling rules, and social structure. *The American Journal of Sociology*, 85(3), 551–575. https://doi.org/10.1086/ 227049

Hochschild, A.R. (1997). *The Time Bind: When Work Becomes Home and Home Becomes Work*. Metropolitan Books.

Hochschild, A.R. (2003 [1983]). *The Managed Heart: Commercialization of Human Feeling* (2nd edn). University of California Press.

Hofstede, G. (1980). *Culture's Consequences: International Differences in Work-Related Values*. SAGE.

Holmes, M. (2010). The emotionalization of reflexivity. *Sociology*, 44(1), 139–154. https://doi.org/10.1177/0038038509351616

Honkasalo, M.-L. (2018). Guest editor's introduction: Vulnerability and inquiring into relationality. *Suomen Antropologi* [*Journal of the Finnish Anthropological Society*], 43(3), 1–21. https://doi.org/10.30676/jfas. v43i3.82725

Honneth, A. (2004). Organized self-realization: Some paradoxes of individualization. *European Journal of Social Theory*, 7(4), 463–478. https:// doi.org/10.1177/1368431004046703

Horwitz, A.V. (2003). *Creating Mental Illness*. University of Chicago Press.

Horwitz, A.V. (2009). An overview of sociological perspectives on the definitions, causes, and responses to mental health and illness. In T.L. Scheid and T.N. Brown (eds), *A Handbook for the Study of Mental Health: Social Contexts, Theories, and Systems* (pp 6–19). Cambridge University Press. https://doi.org/10.1017/CBO9780511984945

Hughes, J. (2005). Bringing emotion to work: Emotional intelligence, employee resistance, and the reinvention of character. *Work Employment & Society*, 19(3), 603–625. https://doi.org/10.1177/0950017005055675

Hutcheon, E. and Lashewicz, B. (2014). Theorizing resilience: Critiquing and unbounding a marginalizing concept. *Disability & Society*, 29(9), 1383–1397. https://doi.org/10.1080/09687599.2014.934954

Illouz, E. (2008). *Saving the Modern Soul: Therapy, Emotions, and the Culture of Self-help*. University of California Press.

Imdorf, C. (2010). Emotions in the hiring procedure: How 'gut feelings' rationalize personnel selection decisions. In B. Sieben and Å. Wettergren (eds), *Emotionalizing Organizations and Organizing Emotions* (pp 84–105). Palgrave Macmillan.

Irvine, E. (2021). The role of replication studies in theory building. *Perspectives on Psychological Science*, 16(4), 844–853. https://doi.org/10.1177/1745691620970558

Issakainen, M. (2016). *Youth Depression: Young People's Distress in Relation to the Cultural Conceptions of Depression*. Https://Erepo.Uef.Fi/Bitstream/Handle/123456789/16971/Urn_isbn_978-952-61-2229-8.Pdf?Sequence=1&isAllowed=y. https://erepo.uef.fi/bitstream/handle/123456789/16971/urn_isbn_978-952-61-2229-8.pdf?sequence=1&isAllowed=y

Jackson, S.E. and Maslach, C. (1982). After-effects of job-related stress: Families as victims. *Journal of Organizational Behavior*, 3(1), 63–77. https://doi.org/10.1002/job.4030030106

Järvensivu, A., Väänänen, A., Kuokkanen, A. and Turtiainen, J. (2018). Mistä syntyy mielenterveysdiagnoosi? [How mental health diagnosis is constructed?]. *Yhteiskuntapolitiikka* [*Journal of Social Policy*], 83(1), 29–39.

Järvisalo, J., Raitasalo, R., Salminen, J.K., Klaukka, T. and Kinnunen, E. (2005). Depression and other mental disorders, sickness absenteeism and work disability pensions in Finland. In J. Järvisalo, B. Anderson, W. Boedeker and I. Houtman (eds), *Mental Disorders as a Major Challenge in Prevention of Work Disability: Experiences in Finland, Germany, the Netherlands and Sweden* (pp 27–59). KELA.

Jenkins, J.H. (2012). The anthropology of psychopharmacology: Commentary on contributions to the analysis of pharmaceutical self and imaginary. *Culture, Medicine and Psychiatry*, 36(1), 78–79. https://doi.org/10.1007/s11013-012-9248-0

Jenkins, J.H. (2015). *Extraordinary Conditions: Culture and Experience in Mental Illness*. University of California Press.

Jones, F., Bright, J. and Clow, A. (2001). *Stress: Myth, Theory and Research*. Prentice Hall.

Jones, R. (2014). The best of times, the worst of times: Social work and its moment. *The British Journal of Social Work*, 44(3), 485–502. https://doi.org/10.1093/bjsw/bcs157

Jorm, A.F. (2000). Mental health literacy: Public knowledge and beliefs about mental disorders. *British Journal of Psychiatry*, 177, 396–401.

Jorm, A.F., Korten, A.E., Rodgers, B., Pollitt, P., Jacomb, P.A., Christensen, H. and Jiao, Z. (1997). Belief systems of the general public concerning the appropriate treatments for mental disorders. *Social Psychiatry and Psychiatric Epidemiology*, 32(8), 468–473. https://doi.org/10.1007/BF00789141

Jorm, A.F., Angermeyer, M. and Katschnig, H. (2000). Public knowledge of and attitudes to mental disorders: A limiting factor in the optimal use of treatment services. In G. Andrews and S. Henderson (eds), *Unmet Need in Psychiatry: Problems, Resources, Responses* (pp 399–413). Cambridge University Press. https://doi.org/10.1017/CBO9780511543562

Jorm, A.F., Barney, L.J., Christensen, H., Highet, N.J., Kelly, C.M. and Kitchener, B.A. (2006). Research on mental health literacy: What we know and what we still need to know. *Australian and New Zealand Journal of Psychiatry*, 40(1), 3–5. https://doi.org/10.1080/j.1440-1614.2006.01734.x

Joukamaa, M. (2002). Sosiaalipsykiatria [Social psychiatry]. In U. Lepola (ed), *Psykiatria [Psychiatry]*. WSOY.

Julkunen, R. (2003). Hiipivä ja ryömivä – pääoma valtaamassa hyvinvointivaltiota [Capital is occupying welfare state]. In H. Melin and J. Nikula (eds), *Yhteiskunnallinen muutos [Societal Change]* (pp 181–192). Vastapaino.

Julkunen, R. (2008). *Uuden työn paradoksit: Keskusteluja 2000-luvun työprosess(e)ista [New Paradoxes of Work: Discussions about 21st-Century Work Processes]*. Vastapaino.

Kaila, M. (1942). Uber die Durchschinittshäufigkeit der Geisteskrankheiten und des Schwachsinns in Finnland [About the average incidence of mental illness and mental deficiency in Finland]. *Acta Psychiatrica Scandinavica*, 17(1), 47–67. https://doi.org/10.1111/j.1600-0447.1942.tb06767.x

Kalleberg, A.L. (2009). Precarious work, insecure workers: Employment relations in transition. *American Sociological Review*, 74(1), 1–22. https://doi.org/10.1177/000312240907400101

Kalleberg, A.L. (2011). *Good Jobs, Bad Jobs: The Rise of Polarized and Precarious Employment Systems in the United States, 1970s–2000s* (pp xvi–xvi). Russell Sage Foundation. https://doi.org/10.7758/9781610447478

Kalleberg, A.L. (2018). *Precarious Lives: Job Insecurity and Well-Being in Rich Democracies*. John Wiley & Sons.

Kantola, A. (2002). *Markkinakuri ja managerivalta: Poliittinen hallinta Suomen 1990-luvun talouskriisissä [Market Discipline and Managerial Power: Political Governing in the Finnish Economic Crisis in the 1990s]*. Loki-kirjat.

Kantola, A. (2014). *Matala valta [Low Power]*. Vastapaino.

Kaplan, G.A. (2004). What's wrong with social epidemiology, and how can we make it better? *Epidemiologic Reviews*, 26(1), 124–135. https://doi.org/10.1093/epirev/mxh010

Karasek, R.A. (1979). Job demands, job decision latitude, and mental strain: Implications for job redesign. *Administrative Science Quarterly*, 24(2), 285–308. https://doi.org/10.2307/2392498

Karasek, R. and Theorell, T. (1990). *Healthy Work: Stress, Productivity, and the Reconstruction of Working Life*. Basic Books.

Karp, D.A. (2017). *Speaking of Sadness: Depression, Disconnection, and the Meanings of Illness*. Oxford University Press.

Kassarjian, W.M. (1962). A study of Riesman's theory of social character. *Sociometry*, 25(3), 213–230. https://doi.org/10.2307/2786125

Katz, D. and Kahn, R.L. (1966). *The Social Psychology of Organizations*. John Wiley & Sons.

Kauppinen, T., Uuksulainen, S., Saalo, A. and Mäkinen, I. (2013). Trends of occupational exposure to chemical agents in Finland in 1950–2020. *The Annals of Occupational Hygiene*, 57(5), 593–609. https://doi.org/10.1093/annhyg/mes090

Kawakami, N., Araki, S. and Kawashima, M. (1990). Effects of job stress on occurrence of major depression in Japanese industry: A case-control study nested in a cohort study. *Journal of Occupational Medicine*, 32(8), 722–725.

Kelly, M.G.E. (2013). Foucault, subjectivity, and technologies of the self. In C. Falzon, T. O'Leary and J. Sawicki (eds), *A Companion to Foucault* (pp 510–525). Blackwell.

Kerr, C., Dunlop, J.T., Harbison, F. and Myers, C.A. (1962). *Industrialism and Industrial Man: The Problems of Labour and Management in Economic Growth*. Harvard University Press.

Kettunen, P. (1994). *Suojelu, suoritus, subjekti: Työsuojelu teollistuvan Suomen yhteiskunnallisissa ajattelu- ja toimintatavoissa* [*Protection, Output, Subject: Occupational Protection in Industrializing Finland's Societal Methods of Thinking and Acting*]. SHS.

Kettunen, P. (2006). The tension between the social and the economic: A historical perspective on a welfare state. In J. Ojala, J. Eloranta and J. Jalava (eds), *The Road to Prosperity: An Economic History of Finland* (pp 285–313). SKS.

Keyriläinen, M. (2021). *Työolobarometri 2020* [*Working Life Barometer 2020*]. Työ- ja elinkeinoministeriö [Ministry of Economic Affairs and Employment of Finland]. https://julkaisut.valtioneuvosto.fi/handle/10024/163200

Kincaid, H. and Sullivan, J.A. (2014). *Classifying Psychopathology: Mental Kinds and Natural Kinds*. The MIT Press. https://doi.org/10.7551/mitpress/8942.001.0001

King, D.B. (2009). The Roman period and the Middle Ages. In D.B. King, W. Viney and W.D. Woody (eds), *A History of Psychology: Ideas and Context* (pp 70–71). Pearson.

Kinnunen, A. (2020a). *Johtolankoja hulluuteen: Tutkimus mielen sairastamiseen kytkeytyvistä kulttuurisista käsityksistä* [*Clues to Madness: Research About Cultural Views Connected to Mental Illness*] [Doctoral Dissertation]. Suomen kansantietouden tutkijain seura [Folkloristic Researchers in Finland].

Kinnunen, A. (2020b). Mielen sairastaminen ja poikkeavuuden rajat: Lectio praecursoria Itä-Suomen yliopistossa 4.12.2020 [Mental illness and atypical limits: lectio praecursoria in University of Eastern-Finland]. *Elore*, 27(2), Article 2. https://doi.org/10.30666/elore.100392

Kinnunen-Amaroso, M. and Liira, J. (2014). Work-related stress management by Finnish enterprises. *Industrial Health*, 52(3), 216–224. https://doi.org/10.2486/indhealth.2013-0178

Kira, M. (2003). *Byrokratian jälkeen: Kohti uudistavaa työtä ja kestävää työjärjestelmäkehitystä* [*After the Bureaucracy: Towards Development of Regenerative and Sustainable Work Systems*]. Työministeriö [Ministry of Labour].

Kivistö, S., Turtiainen, J. and Väänänen, A. (2014). Suojelusta työhyvinvointiin: Työntekijyyden ja työympäristön rajojen muutos työturvallisuuden lainvalmistelussa [Change from the protection to well-being at work: Changed workership and the boundaries of work environment in the occupational safety-lawmaking process]. In A. Väänänen and J. Turtiainen (eds), *Suomalainen työntekijyys 1945–2013* [*Finnish Employment from 1945 to 2013*] (pp 189–226). Vastapaino.

Kjaerulff, J. (2015). *Flexible Capitalism: Exchange and Ambiguity at Work*. Berghahn Books.

Klein, D.N., Kotov, R. and Bufferd, S.J. (2011). Personality and depression: Explanatory models and review of the evidence. *Annual Review of Clinical Psychology*, 7(1), 269–295. https://doi.org/10.1146/annurev-clinpsy-032210-104540

Kleinman, A. and Becker, A.E. (1998). 'Sociosomatics': The contributions of anthropology to psychosomatic medicine. *Psychosomatic Medicine*, 60(4), 389–393. https://doi.org/10.1097/00006842-199807000-00001

Kleinman, A., Eisenberg, L. and Good, B. (1978). Culture, illness, and care: Clinical lessons from anthropologic and cross-cultural research. *Annals of Internal Medicine*, 88(2), 251–258. https://doi.org/10.7326/0003-4819-88-2-251

Kleinman, A., Eisenberg, L. and Good, B. (1985). *Culture and Depression: Studies in the Anthropology and Cross-Cultural Psychiatry of Affect and Disorder*. University of California Press.

Kleinman, A., Mechanic, D., Osterweis, M. and Institute of Medicine (US) Committee on Pain, Disability, and Chronic Illness Behavior (1987). *Pain and Disability: Clinical, Behavioral, and Public Policy Perspectives*. National Academy Press.

Knights, D. and Willmott, H. (1995). Culture and control in an insurance company. *Studies in Cultures, Organizations and Societies*, 1, 29–46. https://doi.org/10.1080/10245289508523444

Knottnerus, J.D. (2010). Collective events, rituals, and emotions. In S.R. Thye and E.J. Lawler (eds), *Advances in Group Processes* (Vol 27, pp 39–61). Emerald Group Publishing Limited. https://doi.org/10.1108/S0882-6145(2010)0000027005

Knudsen, A.K., Allebeck, P., Tollånes, M.C., Skogen, J.C., Iburg, K.M., McGrath, J.J. et al (2019). Life expectancy and disease burden in the Nordic countries: Results from the global burden of diseases, injuries, and risk factors study 2017. *The Lancet*, 4(12), e658–e669. https://doi.org/10.1016/S2468-2667(19)30224-5

Koenen, K.C., Moffitt, T.E., Roberts, A.L., Martin, L.T., Kubzansky, L., Harrington, H., Poulton, R. and Caspi, A. (2009). Childhood IQ and adult mental disorders: A test of the cognitive reserve hypothesis. *The American Journal of Psychiatry*, 166(1), 50–57. https://doi.org/10.1176/appi.ajp.2008.08030343

Kokkinen, L., Kouvonen, A., Buscariolli, A., Koskinen, A., Varje, P. and Väänänen, A. (2019). Human service work and long-term sickness absence due to mental disorders: A prospective study of gender-specific patterns in 1,466,100 employees. *Annals of Epidemiology*, 31, 57–61. https://doi.org/10.1016/j.annepidem.2018.12.006

Kokkinen, L., Gluschkoff, K., Kausto, J., Selinheimo, S., Appelqvist-Schmidlechner, K., Koponen, P. and Väänänen, A. (2023). Occupational grade, mental distress, and the use of psychotherapy. *Journal of Primary Care & Community Health*, 14, 21501319231199960. https://doi.org/10.1177/21501319231199958

Koppes, L.L. (ed). (2007). *Historical Perspectives in Industrial and Organizational Psychology*. Erlbaum.

Kornhauser, A. (1962). Toward an assessment of the mental health of factory workers: A Detroit study. *Human Organization*, 21(1), 43–46.

Kornhauser, A.W. and Reid, O.M. (1965). *Mental Health of the Industrial Worker: A Detroit Study*. John Wiley & Sons.

Kortteinen, M. (1992). *Kunnian kenttä: Suomalainen palkkatyö kulttuurisena muotona* [*Finnish Wagework as Cultural Form*]. Hanki ja Jää.

Kosonen, P. (1998). *Pohjoismaiset mallit murroksessa* [*The Nordic Welfare Models in Change*]. Vastapaino.

Kotchemidova, C. (2005). From good cheer to 'drive-by smiling': A social history of cheerfulness. *Journal of Social History*, 39(1), 5–37.

Kouvonen, A., Koskinen, A., Varje, P., Kokkinen, L., Vogli, R.D. and Väänänen, A. (2014). National trends in main causes of hospitalization: A multi-cohort register study of the Finnish working-age population, 1976–2010. *PLOS ONE*, 9(11), e112314. https://doi.org/10.1371/journal.pone.0112314

Kugelmann, R. (1992). *Stress: The Nature and History of Engineered Grief*. Praeger.

Kunda, G. and Ailon-Souday, G. (2006). Managers, markets, and ideologies: Design and devotion revisited. In S. Ackroyd, R. Batt, P. Thompson and P.S. Tolbert (eds), *The Oxford Handbook of Work and Organization* (pp 200–219). Oxford University Press. https://doi.org/10.1093/oxfordhb/9780199299249.003.0011

Kuokkanen, A., Varje, P. and Väänänen, A. (2013). Transformation of the Finnish employee ideal in job advertisements from 1944 to 2009. *Acta Sociologica*, 56(3), 213–226. https://doi.org/10.1177/0001699313477871

Kuokkanen, A., Varje, P. and Väänänen, A. (2020). Struggle over employees psychological well-being. The politization and depolitization of the debate on employee mental health in the Finnish insurance sector. *Management & Organizational History*, 15(3), 252–272. https://doi.org/10.1080/17449359.2020.1845741

Kury, P. (2017). Neurasthenia and managerial disease in Germany and America: Transnational ties and national characteristics in the field of exhaustion 1880–1960. In S. Neckel, A.K. Schaffner and G. Wagner (eds), *Burnout, Fatigue, Exhaustion: An Interdisciplinary Perspective on a Modern Affliction* (pp 51–73). Springer International Publishing.

Laaksonen, M. and Blomgren, J. (2020). The level and development of unemployment before disability retirement: A retrospective study of Finnish disability retirees and their controls. *International Journal of Environmental Research and Public Health*, 17(5), 1756. https://doi.org/10.3390/ijerph17051756

Labaree, D.F. (2000). On the nature of teaching and teacher education: Difficult practices that look easy. *Journal of Teacher Education*, 51(3), 228–233. https://doi.org/10.1177/0022487100051003011

Lahelma, E., Laaksonen, M., Martikainen, P., Rahkonen, O. and Sarlio-Lähteenkorva, S. (2006). Multiple measures of socioeconomic circumstances and common mental disorders. *Social Science & Medicine*, 63(5), 1383–1399. https://doi.org/10.1016/j.socscimed.2006.03.027

Land, K.C. (1975). Theories, models and indicators of social change. *International Social Science Journal*, 27(1), 7–37.

Lane, C. (2007). *Shyness: How Normal Behavior Became a Sickness*. Yale University Press.

Laqueur, T. (1992). *Making Sex: Body and Gender from the Greeks to Freud*. Harvard University Press.

Lash, S. and Urry, J. (1987). *The End of Organized Capitalism*. Polity Press.

Lash, S. and Urry, J. (2013). Book review symposium: Response to reviewers of *The End of Organized Capitalism*. *Work, Employment & Society*, 27(3), 542–546. https://doi.org/10.1177/0950017013479687

Launonen, L. (2000). *Eettinen kasvatusajattelu suomalaisen koulun pedagogisissa teksteissä 1860-luvulta 1990-luvulle* [*Ethical Thinking in Finnish School's Pedagogical Texts from the 1860s to the 1990s*] [Doctoral Dissertation]. University of Jyväskylä.

Lazonick, W. and O'Sullivan, M. (2000). Maximizing shareholder value: A new ideology for corporate governance. *Economy and Society*, 29(1), 13–35. https://doi.org/10.1080/030851400360541

Lee, G. and Wrench, J. (1987). Race and gender dimensions of the youth labor market: From apprenticeship to YTS. In R. Loveridge (ed), *The Manufacture of Disadvantage: Stigma and Social Closure* (pp 83–99). Open University Press.

Lehmuskoski, K., Mattila-Holappa, P., Juvonen-Posti, P. and Väänänen, A. (2022). Mielenterveyden toimijahahmot: Laadullinen tutkimus nuorista työntekijöistä kuntasektorilla [Social characters of mental health: A qualitative study of young employees in the municipal sector]. *Kuntoutus* [*Rehabilitation*], 45(4), Article 4. https://doi.org/10.37451/kuntou tus.125397

Lehtonen, M. and Koivunen, A. (2010). Kansalainen minä: Median ihannesubjektit ja suostumuksen tuottaminen [Citizen me: The ideal subjects of media and the production of consent]. In P. Pietikäinen (ed), *Valta Suomessa* [*Dominance in Finland*] (pp 229–250). Gaudeamus.

Leiman, M. (1998). Words as intersubjective mediators in psychotherapeutic discourse: The presence of hidden voices in patient utterances. In M. Lähteenmäki and H. Dufva (eds), *Dialogues on Bakhtin: Interdisciplinary Readings* (pp 106–117). Centre for Applied Language Studies. https://jyx. jyu.fi/handle/123456789/36968

Lerner, J. and Rivkin-Fish, M. (2021). On emotionalisation of public domains. *Emotions and Society*, 3(1), 3–14. https://doi.org/10.1332/26316 9021X16149420135743

Levä, I. (2021). *Toimihenkilöt neuvottelupöydässä: Järjestöt työmarkkinoiden taitekohdissa 1945–2015* [*Organisations in Turning Points of Labour Markets from 1945 to 2015*]. Gaudeamus.

Levi, L. (1978). *Society, Stress and Disease. 3, The Productive and Reproductive Age: Male/Female Roles and Relationships*. Oxford Medical Publications.

Levi-Strauss, C. (2009 [1955]). *A World on the Wane*. Kessinger Publishing.

Lewchuk, W., Clarke, M. and de Wolff, A. (2008). Working without commitments: Precarious employment and health. *Work, Employment and Society*, 22(3), 387–406. https://doi.org/10.1177/0950017008093477

Lewin, K. (1938). *The Conceptual Representation and the Measurement of Psychological Forces*. Duke University Press.

Liu, K.-Y., King, M. and Bearman, P.S. (2010). Social influence and the autism epidemic. *The American Journal of Sociology*, 115(5), 1387–1434. https://doi.org/10.1086/651448

Liu, S.X. (1989). Neurasthenia in China: Modern and traditional criteria for its diagnosis. *Culture, Medicine and Psychiatry*, 13(2), 163–186. https:// doi.org/10.1007/BF02220660

Lively, K.J. and Weed, E.A. (2014). Emotion management: Sociological insight into what, how, why, and to what end? *Emotion Review*, 6(3), 202–207. https://doi.org/10.1177/1754073914522864

Loriol, M. (2019). *Stress and Suffering at Work: The Role of Culture and Society*. Springer.

Löyttyniemi, V. (2001). Doctors drifting: Autonomy and career uncertainty in young physicians' stories. *Social Science & Medicine*, 52(2), 227–237. https://doi.org/10.1016/S0277-9536(00)00223-9

Lupton, D. (1998). *The Emotional Self: A Sociocultural Exploration*. SAGE.

Lupton, D. (2016). *The Quantified Self*. John Wiley & Sons.

Luthans, F. (2007). *Psychological Capital: Developing the Human Competitive Edge*. Oxford University Press.

Lyman, S.M. (1989). *The Seven Deadly Sins: Society and Evil*. Rowman & Littlefield.

Lysaker, O. (2014). Humanity in times of crisis: Hannah Arendt's political existentialism. In G. Fløistad (ed), *Philosophy of Justice* (pp 293–310). Springer. https://doi.org/10.1007/978-94-017-9175-5_17

MacCormack, P. (2020). *The Ahuman Manifesto: Activism for the End of the Anthropocene*. Bloomsbury Publishing.

Mackenbach, J.P. (1994). The epidemiologic transition theory. *Journal of Epidemiology and Community Health*, 48(4), 329–331. https://doi.org/10.1136/jech.48.4.329-a

Madsen, I.E.H., Nyberg, S.T., Magnusson Hanson, L.L., Ferrie, J.E., Ahola, K., Alfredsson, L. et al (2017). Job strain as a risk factor for clinical depression: Systematic review and meta-analysis with additional individual participant data. *Psychological Medicine*, 47(8), 1342–1356. https://doi.org/10.1017/S003329171600355X

Madsen, O.J. (2018). *The Psychologization of Society: On the Unfolding of the Therapeutic in Norway*. Routledge.

Madsen, O.J. (2021). *Deconstructing Scandinavia's 'Achievement Generation': A Youth Mental Health Crisis?* Palgrave Macmillan.

Mai, Q. (2017). Precarious work in Europe: Assessing cross-national differences and institutional determinants of work precarity in 32 European countries. In A. Kalleberg and S.P. Vallas (eds) *Precarious Work (Research in the Sociology of Work*, Vol 31) (pp 273–206). Emerald Publishing Limited.

Manderscheid, R.W., Ryff, C.D., Freeman, E.J., McKnight-Eily, L.R., Dhingra, S. and Strine, T.W. (2010). Evolving definitions of mental illness and wellness. *Preventing Chronic Disease*, 7(1), A19.

Mannevuo, M. (2020). *Ihmiskone töissä: Sotienjälkeinen Suomi tehokkuutta tavoittelemassa* [*Human Machine at Work: Post WWII Finland Seeking Efficiency*]. Gaudeamus.

Marcus, S.C. and Olfson, M. (2010). National trends in the treatment for depression from 1998 to 2007. *Archives of General Psychiatry*, 67, 1265–1273. https://doi.org/10.1001/archgenpsychiatry.2010.151

Marmot, M.G. and Wilkinson, R.G. (eds). (2006). *Social Determinants of Health*. Oxford University Press.

Marques, T.P. (2018). Illness and the politics of social suffering: Towards a critical research agenda in health and science studies. *Revista Crítica de Ciências Sociais, Número especial*, 141–164. https://doi.org/10.4000/rccs.7763

Martimo, K.-P. and Mäkitalo, J. (2014). *The Status of Occupational Health Services in Finland and the Role of the Finnish Institute of Occupational Health in the Development of Occupational Health Services*. Finnish Institute of Occupational Health. https://www.julkari.fi/handle/10024/135062

Maslow, A.H. (1968). *Toward a Psychology of Being* (2nd edn). Van Nostrand.

Mauss, M. (1973 [1934]). Techniques of the body. *Economy and Society*, 2(1), 70–88. https://doi.org/10.1080/03085147300000003

Mazmanian, M., Orlikowski, W.J. and Yates, J. (2013). The autonomy paradox: The implications of mobile email devices for knowledge professionals. *Organization Science*, 24(5), 1337–1357. https://doi.org/10.1287/orsc.1120.0806

McCarthy, E.D. (2002). The emotions: Senses of the modern self. *Österreichische Zeitschrift Für Soziologie*, 27(2), 30–49.

McDaid, D. (2008). *Mental Health in Workplace Settings*. European Communities.

McDonald, M. and O'Callaghan, J. (2008). Positive psychology: A Foucauldian critique. *The Humanistic Psychologist*, 36(2), 127–142. https://doi.org/10.1080/08873260802111119

McDovell, L., Batnitzky, A. and Dyer, S. (2009). Precarious work and economic migration: Emerging immigrant divisions of labour in Greater London's service sector. *International Journal of Urban and Regional Research*, 33(1), 3–25. https://doi.org/10.1111/j.1468-2427.2009.00831.x

McKee, M., Legido-Quigley, H. and Piot, P. (2013). Trends in life expectancy in Europe: One big explanation or many small ones? *European Journal of Epidemiology*, 28(3), 203–204. https://doi.org/10.1007/s10654-013-9778-y

McKendrick, N. (1961). Josiah Wedgwood and factory discipline. *The Historical Journal*, 4(1), 30–55.

McKeon, P. and Carrick, S. (1991). Public attitudes to depression: A national survey. *Irish Journal of Psychological Medicine*, 8(2), 116–121. https://doi.org/10.1017/S0790966700015020

McKinlay, J.B. and Marceau, L.D. (2002). The end of the golden age of doctoring. *International Journal of Health Services*, 32(2), 379–416. https://doi.org/10.2190/JL1D-21BG-PK2N-J0KD

McLaughlin, K.G. (2011). *Surviving Identity Vulnerability and the Psychology of Recognition*. Routledge.

McWhinney, W.R., Adelman, S.R. and Kornhauser, A. (1966). Mental health of the industrial worker: An analysis and review. *Human Organization*, 25(2), 180–182.

Mead, G.H. (2015). *Mind, Self, and Society: The Definitive Edition.* Edited by D.R. Huebner, H. Joas and C.W. Morris. University of Chicago Press.

Mercer, A. (2014). *Infections, Chronic Disease, and the Epidemiological Transition: A New Perspective.* University of Rochester Press.

Merton, R.K. (1968). *Social Theory and Social Structure.* The Free Press.

Meslé, F. and Vallin, J. (2017). The end of East–West divergence in European life expectancies? An introduction to the special issue. *European Journal of Population*, 33(5), 615–627. https://doi.org/10.1007/s10680-017-9452-2

Metzl, J. (2003). *Prozac on the Couch: Prescribing Gender in the Era of Wonder Drugs.* Duke University Press.

Meyer, J.W. and Jepperson, R.L. (2000). The 'actors' of modern society: The cultural construction of social agency. *Sociological Theory*, 18(1), 100–120. https://doi.org/10.1111/0735-2751.00090

Michel, J.S., Kotrba, L.M., Mitchelson, J.K., Clark, M.A. and Baltes, B.B. (2011). Antecedents of work-family conflict: A meta-analytic review. *Journal of Organizational Behavior*, 32(5), 689–725. https://doi.org/10.1002/job.695

Miller, P. and Rose, N. (2008). Production, identity and democracy. In P. Miller and N. Rose (eds), *Governing the Present. Administering Economic, Social and Personal Life* (pp 173–198). Polity Press.

Mills, C.W. (1959). *The Sociological Imagination.* Oxford University Press.

Milner, A., Kavanagh, A., King, T. and Currier, D. (2018). The influence of masculine norms and occupational factors on mental health: Evidence from the baseline of the Australian longitudinal study on male health. *American Journal of Men's Health*, 12(4), 696–705. https://doi.org/10.1177/1557988317752607

Modell, H., Cliff, W., Michael, J., McFarland, J., Wenderoth, M.P. and Wright, A. (2015). A physiologist's view of homeostasis. *Advances in Physiology Education*, 39(4), 259–266. https://doi.org/10.1152/advan.00107.2015

Mojtabai, R. (2008). Increase in antidepressant medication in the US adult population between 1990 and 2003. *Psychotherapy and Psychosomatics*, 77(2), 83–92. https://doi.org/10.1159/000112885

Moloney, M.E. (2017). 'Sometimes, it's easier to write the prescription': Physician and patient accounts of the reluctant medicalisation of sleeplessness. *Sociology of Health & Illness*, 39(3), 333–348. https://doi.org/10.1111/1467-9566.12485

Mookherjee, M. (2005). Affective citizenship: Feminism, postcolonialism and the politics of recognition. *Critical Review of International Social and Political Philosophy*, 8(1), 31–50. https://doi.org/10.1080/1369823042000335830

Morant, N. (2006). Social representations and professional knowledge: The representation of mental illness among mental health practitioners. *The British Journal of Social Psychology*, 45(Pt 4), 817–838. https://doi.org/10.1348/014466605x81036

Moriarty, D.G., Zack, M.M., Holt, J.B., Chapman, D.P. and Safran, M.A. (2009). Geographic patterns of frequent mental distress: U.S. adults, 1993–2001 and 2003–2006. *American Journal of Preventive Medicine*, 36(6), 497–505. https://doi.org/10.1016/j.amepre.2009.01.038

Morris, J.A. and Feldman, D.C. (1997). Managing emotions in the workplace. *Journal of Managerial Issues*, 9(3), 257–274.

Morton, T. (2016). *Dark Ecology: For a Logic of Future Coexistence*. Columbia University Press

Moser, S. and Schlechtriemen, T. (2019). Social figures: Between societal experience and sociological diagnosis. *Halshs-01972078*. https://shs.hal.science/halshs-01972078/document

Moulier-Boutang, Y. (2011). *Cognitive Capitalism*. Polity.

Munro, V.E. and Scoular, J. (2012). Abusing vulnerability? Contemporary law and policy responses to sex work in the UK. *Feminist Legal Studies*, 20(3), 189–206. https://doi.org/10.1007/s10691-012-9213-x

Muntaner, C. and Chung, H. (2007). Class relations, economic inequality and mental health: Why social class matters to the sociology of mental health. In W.R. Avison, J.D. McLeod and B.A. Pescosolido (eds), *Mental Health, Social Mirror* (pp 127–142). Springer.

Murray, H.A. (1938). *Explorations in Personality*. Oxford University Press.

Murray, K. (1989). The construction of identity in the narratives of romance and comedy. In J. Shotter and K.J. Gergen (eds), *Texts of Identity* (pp 176–205). SAGE.

Murray, M., Pullman, D. and Rodgers, T.H. (2003). Social representations of health and illness among 'baby-boomers' in Eastern Canada. *Journal of Health Psychology*, 8(5), 485–499. https://doi.org/10.1177/1359105303 0085002

Näring, G., Briët, M. and Brouwers, A. (2006). Beyond demand-control: Emotional labour and symptoms of burnout in teachers. *Work and Stress*, 20(4), 303–315. https://doi.org/10.1080/02678370601065182

Neckel, S., Schaffner, A.K. and Wagner, G. (2017). *Burnout, Fatigue, Exhaustion: An Interdisciplinary Perspective on a Modern Affliction*. Springer.

Negele, A., Kaufhold, J., Kallenbach, L. and Leuzinger-Bohleber, M. (2015). Childhood trauma and its relation to chronic depression in adulthood. *Depression Research and Treatment*, 1–11. https://doi.org/10.1155/2015/650804

Nehring, D., Madsen, O.J., Cabanas, E., Mills, C. and Kerrigan, D. (eds). (2020). *The Routledge International Handbook of Global Therapeutic Cultures*. Routledge.

Neufeld, S.A.S. (2022). The burden of young people's mental health conditions in Europe: No cause for complacency. *The Lancet Regional Health – Europe*, 16, 100364. https://doi.org/10.1016/j.lanepe.2022.100364

Neugarten, B.L. (1973). Personality change in late life: A developmental perspective. In C. Eisdorfer and M.P. Lawton (eds), *The Psychology of Adult Development and Aging* (pp 311–335). American Psychological Association. https://doi.org/10.1037/10044-000

Newton, T. (1995). Retheorizing stress and emotion: Labour process theory, Foucault and Elias. In T. Newton, J. Handy and S. Fineman (eds), *'Managing' Stress: Emotion and Power at Work* (pp 58–82). SAGE.

Newton, T. (1998). Theorizing subjectivity in organizations: The failure of Foucauldian studies? *Organization Studies*, 19(3), 415–447. https://doi.org/10.1177/017084069801900303

Newton, T. (2009). Organizations and the natural environment. In M. Alvesson, T. Bridgman and H. Willmott (eds), *The Oxford Handbook of Critical Management Studies* (pp 125–143). Cambridge University Press.

Newton, T. (2022). Psychology: Where history, culture, and biology meet. *Theory & Psychology*, 09593543221131782. https://doi.org/10.1177/09593543221131782

Newton, T., Deetz, S. and Reed, M. (2011). Responses to social constructionism and critical realism in organization studies. *Organization Studies*, 32(1), 7–26. https://doi.org/10.1177/0170840610394289

Newton, T., Luca, R., Slutskaya, N. and Game, A. (2022). The 'narrow self'? Developing a critical-historical work psychology. *Applied Psychology*, 72. https://doi.org/10.1111/apps.12421

Niemi, A.-M. and Mietola, R. (2017). Between hopes and possibilities. (Special) educational paths, agency and subjectivities. *Scandinavian Journal of Disability Research*, 19(3), 218–229. https://doi.org/10.1080/15017419.2016.1239588

Nordberg, S. (2022). *Itsensä kehittäminen ja toteuttaminen yksilöllistävän vallan ilmiönä. Aikakauslehtianalyysi vuosilta 1947–2017* [*Personal Development and Fulfillment as a Phenomena of Individualizing Power. Journal Analysis from 1947 to 2017*] [Master's Thesis]. University of Helsinki.

Nyman, H. and Kiviniemi, M. (2015). *Katsaus eläketurvaan vuonna 2014* [*Overview to Pension Security in Finland 2014*] Finnish Centre for Pensions. https://www.julkari.fi/handle/10024/129340

Nyman, H. and Kiviniemi, M. (2018). *Katsaus eläketurvaan vuonna 2017* [*Overview to Pension Security in Finland 2017*] (06/2018; Eläketurvakeskuksen tilastoja). Finnish Centre for Pensions. https://www.julkari.fi/handle/10024/136579

OECD (2010). *Sickness, Disability and Work: Breaking the Barriers: A Synthesis of Findings across OECD Countries*. OECD.

OECD (2015). *Fit Mind, Fit Job: From Evidence to Practice in Mental Health and Work*. OECD. https://www.oecd-ilibrary.org/employment/fit-mind-fit-job_9789264228283-en

OECD (2017). *Technology and Innovation in the Insurance Sector.* OECD Publishing.

Ojala, S., Pyöriä, P. and Riekhoff, A.-J. (2021). Career stability in 14 Finnish industrial employee cohorts in 1988–2015. *Nordic Journal of Working Life Studies*, 11(2). https://doi.org/10.18291/njwls.123167

Oksanen, A. and Turtiainen, J. (2005). A life told in ink: Tattoo narratives and the problem of the self in late modern society. *Auto/Biography*, 13(2), 111–130. https://doi.org/10.1191/0967550705ab021oa

Olakivi, A. (2018). *The Relational Construction of Occupational Agency: Performing Professional and Enterprising Selves in Diversifying Care Work.* University of Helsinki.

Olakivi, A., Kouvonen, A., Koskinen, A., Kemppainen, L., Kokkinen, L. and Väänänen, A. (2023). Sickness absence among migrant and non-migrant care workers in Finland: A register-based follow-up study. *Scandinavian Journal of Public Health*, 14034948231168434. https://doi.org/10.1177/14034948231168434

Olsen, R.K. (2006). A change from leadership (vertical powerstructure) to leadingship (horizontal powerstructure) at work. *The New Workplace Reality Series*. https://www.humiliationstudies.org/documents/OlsenLeadershipLeadingship.pdf

Omran, A.R. (1971). The epidemiologic transition: A theory of the epidemiology of population change. *The Milbank Memorial Fund Quarterly*, 49(4), 509–538. https://doi.org/10.2307/3349375

Orlikowski, W.J. and Yates, J. (2002). It's about time: Temporal structuring in organizations. *Organization Science*, 13(6), 684–700. https://doi.org/10.1287/orsc.13.6.684.501

Patomäki, H. (2007). *Uusliberalismi Suomessa: Lyhyt historia ja tulevaisuuden vaihtoehdot [Neoliberalism in Finland: Short History and the Options for the Future]*. WSOY.

Pattyn, E. (2014). *Holding Up a Sociological Mirror to the Mental Health Treatment Gap* [Dissertation]. Ghent University. http://hdl.handle.net/1854/LU-5688013

Pedriana, N. (2004). Help wanted NOW: Legal resources, the women's movement, and the battle over sex-segregated job advertisements. *Social Problems*, 51(2), 182–201. https://doi.org/10.1525/sp.2004.51.2.182

Pescosolido, B.A., Gardner, C.B. and Lubell, K.M. (1998). How people get into mental health services: Stories of choice, coercion and 'muddling through' from 'first-timers'. *Social Science & Medicine*, 46(2), 275–286. https://doi.org/10.1016/S0277-9536(97)00160-3

Petersen, A.R. and Wilkinson, I. (2008). Health, risk and vulnerability: An introduction. In A.R. Petersen and I. Wilkinson (eds), *Health, Risk and Vulnerability* (pp 1–15). Routledge.

Pierret, J. (1995). The social meanings of health: Paris, the essonne, the herault. In M. Augé and C. Herzlich (eds), *The Meaning of Illness: Anthropology, History and Sociology* (pp 175–206). Harwood Academic Publishers.

Pietikäinen, P. (2013). *Hulluuden historia* [*History of Madness*]. Gaudeamus Helsinki University Press.

Pike, K.M. and Dunne, P.E. (2015). The rise of eating disorders in Asia: A review. *Journal of Eating Disorders*, 3(1), 33–33. https://doi.org/10.1186/s40337-015-0070-2

Pirkola, S. (2019). Mielenterveys valokeilassa – Vihdoinkin! [Mental health in the spotlight – at last!]. *Sosiaalilääketieteellinen Aikakauslehti* [*Finnish Social Medicine Journal*], 56(3), Article 3. https://doi.org/10.23990/sa.84507

Pollock, K. (1988). On the nature of social stress: Production of a modern mythology. *Social Science & Medicine*, 26(3), 381–392. https://doi.org/10.1016/0277-9536(88)90404-2

Porter, R. (1997). *The Greatest Benefit to Mankind: A Medical History of Humanity from Antiquity to the Present*. HarperCollins.

Postle, K. (2002). Working 'between the idea and the reality': Ambiguities and tensions in care managers' work. *British Journal of Social Work*, 32(3), 335–351. https://doi.org/10.1093/bjsw/32.3.335

Prins, R. (2013). Sickness absence and disability: An international perspective. In P. Loisel and J.R. Anema (eds), *Handbook of Work Disability: Prevention and Management* (pp 3–14). Springer. https://doi.org/10.1007/978-1-4614-6214-9_1

Purvanova, R.K. and Muros, J.P. (2010). Gender differences in burnout: A meta-analysis. *Journal of Vocational Behavior*, 77(2), 168–185. https://doi.org/10.1016/j.jvb.2010.04.006

Pyöriä, P. and Ojala, S. (2016). Precarious work and intrinsic job quality: Evidence from Finland, 1984–2013. *The Economic and Labour Relations Review*, 27(3), 349–367. https://doi.org/10.1177/1035304616659190

Pyöriä, P., Melin, H. and Blom, R. (2005). *Knowledge Workers in the Information Society: Evidence from Finland*. Tampere University Press. https://trepo.tuni.fi/handle/10024/68142

Rabinbach, A. (1992). *The Human Motor: Energy, Fatigue, and the Origins of Modernity*. University of California Press.

Rappaport, R.A. (1999). *Ritual and Religion in the Making of Humanity*. Cambridge University Press.

Reamer, F.G. (1998). The evolution of social work ethics. *Social Work*, 43(6), 488–500. https://doi.org/10.1093/sw/43.6.488

Reay, D. (2005). Beyond consciousness? The psychic landscape of social class. *Sociology*, 39(5), 911–928. https://doi.org/10.1177/0038038505058372

Renedo, A., Komporozos-Athanasiou, A. and Marston, C. (2018). Experience as evidence: The dialogic construction of health professional knowledge through patient involvement. *Sociology*, 52(4), 778–795. https://doi.org/10.1177/0038038516682457

Richards, G. (2002). *Putting Psychology in Its Place: A Critical Historical Overview*. Psychology Press.

Riesman, D., Glazer, N. and Denney, R. (1950). *The Lonely Crowd. A Study of the Changing American Character*, Yale University Press.

Rikala, S. (2013). *Työssä uupuvat naiset ja masennus* [*Burnout among Women at Work and Depression*] [PhD Thesis]. Tampereen yliopisto [University of Tampere].

Rikala, S. (2014). Masennus työelämässä [Depression in working life]. *Alusta! Yhteiskunta- ja kulttuuritieteiden verkkolehti* [Platform! Digital Journal of Tampere University]. https://www.tuni.fi/alustalehti/2014/02/18/masennus-tyoelamass

Rimke, H. (2008). The developing science of the mind. In R. Lawson (ed), *Research and Discovery: Landmarks and Pioneers in American Science* (pp 526–529). M.E. Sharpe.

Rimke, H. and Brock, D. (2012). The culture of therapy: Psychocentrism in everyday life. In M. Thomas, A. Martin, R. Raby and D. .Brock (eds), *Power and Everyday Practices* (pp. 182-202) Nelson.

Robinson, M. and Robertson, S. (2014). Challenging the field: Bourdieu and men's health. *Social Theory & Health*, 12(4), 339–360. https://doi.org/10.1057/sth.2014.8

Rönnblad, T., Grönholm, E., Jonsson, J., Koranyi, I., Orellana, C., Kreshpaj, B., Chen, L., Stockfelt, L. and Bodin, T. (2019). Precarious employment and mental health: A systematic review and meta-analysis of longitudinal studies. *Scandinavian Journal of Work, Environment & Health*, 45(5), 429–443. https://doi.org/10.5271/sjweh.3797

Roos, J.P. (1987). *Suomalainen elämä* [*Finnish Life*]. SKS.

Rosa, H. (2003). Social acceleration: Ethical and political consequences of a desynchronized high-speed society. *Constellations*, 10(1), 3–33. https://doi.org/10.1111/1467-8675.00309

Rosa, H. (2019). *Resonance: A Sociology of Our Relationship to the World*. Polity Press.

Rose, N. (1989). Individualizing psychology. In K.J. Gergen and J. Shotter (eds), *Texts of Identity* (pp 119–132). SAGE.

Rose, N. (1996). Identity, genealogy, history. In S. Hall and P. du Gay (eds), *Questions of Cultural Identity* (pp 128–150). SAGE.

Rose, N. (1999). *Governing the Soul: The Shaping of the Private Self*. Free Association Books.

Rose, N. (2007). *Politics of Life Itself: Biomedicine, Power and Subjectivity in the Twenty-First Century*. Princeton University Press.

Rose, N. (2018). *Our Psychiatric Future: The Politics of Mental Health*. Polity.

Rosenberg, C.E. (1992). Introduction. In C.E. Rosenberg and J. Gooden (eds), *Framing Disease: Studies in Cultural History*. Rutgers University Press, pp 179–192.

Rosenberg, C.E. (2006). Contested boundaries: Psychiatry, disease, and diagnosis. *Perspectives in Biology and Medicine*, 49(3), 407–424. https://doi.org/10.1353/pbm.2006.0046

Rudnyckyj, D. (2009). Spiritual economies: Islam and neoliberalism in contemporary Indonesia. *Cultural Anthropology*, 24(1), 104–141. https://doi.org/10.1111/j.1548-1360.2009.00028.x

Ryder, A.G., Yang, J. and Heine, S.J. (2002). Somatization vs. psychologization of emotional distress: A paradigmatic example for cultural psychopathology. *Online Readings in Psychology and Culture*, 10(2). https://doi.org/10.9707/2307-0919.1080

Ryff, C.D. and Singer, B.H. (2013). Know thyself and become what you are: A eudaimonic approach to psychological well-being. In D.F. Antonella (ed), *The Exploration of Happiness* (pp 97–116). Springer Netherlands. https://doi.org/10.1007/978-94-007-5702-8_6

Saastamoinen, M. (2006). Yksilö, riskitietoisuus ja psykokulttuuri [Individual, risk-knowledge and psykoculture]. In P. Rautio and M. Saastamoinen (eds), *Minuus ja identiteetti: Sosiaalipsykologinen ja sosiologinen näkökulma* (pp 136–161). Tampere University Press.

Salmenniemi, S. (2022). *Affect, Alienation, and Politics in Therapeutic Culture: Capitalism on the Skin*. Palgrave Macmillan.

Saltonstall, R. (1993). Healthy bodies, social bodies: Men's and women's concepts and practices of health in everyday life. *Social Science & Medicine*, 36(1), 7–14. https://doi.org/10.1016/0277-9536(93)90300-S

Sassen, S. (1998). *Globalization and Its Discontents*. New Press.

Satka, M. (1994). Sosiaalinen työ: Peräänkatsojamiehestä hoivayrittäjäksi [The evolution of social work in Finland]. In J. Jaakkola, P. Pulma and M. Satka (eds), *Armeliaisuus, yhteisöapu, sosiaaliturva. Suomalaisen sosiaalisen turvan historia* [History of Social Security in Finland] (pp 261–334). Gummerus.

Satka, M. (1995). *Making Social Citizenship: Conceptual Practices from the Finnish Poor Law to Professional Social Work* [Doctoral dissertation]. University of Jyväskylä. https://jyx.jyu.fi/handle/123456789/26927

Sayer, A. (2020). Critiquing – and rescuing – 'character'. *Sociology*, 54(3), 460–481. https://doi.org/10.1177/0038038519892532

Schaffner, A.K. (2017). Pre-modern exhaustion: On melancholia and acedia. In S. Neckel, A.K. Schaffner and G. Wagner (eds), *Burnout, Fatigue, Exhaustion: An Interdisciplinary Perspective on a Modern Affliction* (pp 27–50). Springer.

Schaufeli, W.B. (2017). Burnout: A short socio-cultural history. In S. Neckel, A.K. Schaffner and G. Wagner (eds), *Burnout, Fatigue, Exhaustion: An Interdisciplinary Perspective on a Modern Affliction* (pp 105–128). Springer.

Scheff, T.J. (1967). *Mental Illness and Social Processes*. Harper & Row.

Schippers, M. (2007). Recovering the feminine other: Masculinity, femininity, and gender hegemony. *Theory and Society*, 36(1), 85–102. https://doi.org/10.1007/s11186-007-9022-4

Schmidt, T.R. (2021). 'It's OK to feel': The emotionality norm and its evolution in U.S. print journalism. *Journalism*, 22(5), 1173–1189. https://doi.org/10.1177/1464884920985722

Schnittker, J. (2021). *Unnerved: Anxiety, Social Change, and the Transformation of Modern Mental Health*. Columbia University Press.

Seeck, H. (2008). *Johtamisopit Suomessa: Taylorismista innovaatioteorioihin* [*Management Paradigms in Finland: From Taylorism to the Theories of Innovation*]. Gaudeamus.

Seligman, M.E.P. (2002). *Authentic Happiness: Using the New Positive Psychology to Realize Your Potential for Lasting Fulfillment*. Simon & Schuster.

Seligman, M.E.P. and Csikszentmihalyi, M. (2000). Positive psychology: An introduction. *The American Psychologist*, 55(1), 5–14. https://doi.org/10.1037/0003-066X.55.1.5

Selinheimo, S., Gluschkoff, K., Kausto, J., Turunen, J., Koskinen, A. and Väänänen, A. (2023). The association of sociodemographic characteristics with work disability trajectories during and following long-term psychotherapy: A longitudinal register study. *Social Psychiatry and Psychiatric Epidemiology*. https://doi.org/10.1007/s00127-023-02523-y

Semetsky, I. (2008). *Nomadic Education: Variations on a Theme by Deleuze and Guattari*. Sense Publishers.

Sennett, R. (1998). *The Corrosion of Character: The Personal Consequences of Work in the New Capitalism*. Norton.

Shields, S.A. (2002). *Speaking from the Heart: Gender and the Social Meaning of Emotion*. Cambridge University Press.

Shilling, C. (2002). Culture, the 'sick role' and the consumption of health. *The British Journal of Sociology*, 53(4), 621–638. https://doi.org/10.1080/0007131022000021515

Shilling, C. (2003). *The Body and Social Theory*. SAGE.

Shilling, C. and Mellor, P.A. (2022). Social character, interdependence, and the dualities of other-directedness. *The British Journal of Sociology*, 73(1), 125–138. https://doi.org/10.1111/1468-4446.12902

Shiraev, E.B. and Levy, D.A. (2020). *Cross-Cultural Psychology: Critical Thinking and Contemporary Applications*. Routledge.

Shorter, E. (1997). *A History of Psychiatry: From the Era of the Asylum to the Age of Prozac*. John Wiley & Sons.

Shorter, E. (2013). *How Everyone Became Depressed: The Rise and Fall of the Nervous Breakdown*. Oxford University Press.

Siegrist, J. (1996). Adverse health effects of high-effort/low-reward conditions. *Journal of Occupational Health Psychology*, 1(1), 27–41. https://doi.org/10.1037/1076-8998.1.1.27

Siegrist, J. and Marmot, M. (eds). (2006). *Social Inequalities in Health: New Evidence and Policy Implications* (Illustrated edition). Oxford University Press.

Siltala, J. (2007). *Työelämän huonontumisen lyhyt historia: Muutokset hyvinvointivaltioiden ajasta globaaliin hyperkilpailuun* [*The Short History of Worsening of Work: Changes from the Time of Welfare State to Global Hyberrace*] (Renewed edition). Otava.

Silvonen, J. (2015). Toiminta ja suhteet – Neljä fragmenttia toimijuudesta [Behaviour and relations – four fragments of human agency]. In P.A. Kauppila, J. Silvonen and M. Vanhalakkaruoho (eds), *Toimijuus, ohjaus, elämänkulku* (pp 3–15). University of Eastern Finland.

Simmel, G. (1950 [1903]). The metropolis and mental life. In *The Sociology of Georg Simmel* (pp 409–424). Free Press.

Simola, H. (1998). Constructing a school-free pedagogy: Decontextualization of Finnish state educational discourse. *Journal of Curriculum Studies*, 30(3), 339–356. https://doi.org/10.1080/002202798183648

Simons, R.C. (2003). Littlewood, Roland. *Pathologies of the West: An Anthropology of Mental Illness in Europe and America. Journal of the Royal Anthropological Institute*, 9(3), 590.

Sippola, M. (2012). The restructuring of the Nordic labour process and the variegated status of workers in the labour market. *Competition & Change*, 16(3), 243–260. https://doi.org/10.1179/1024529412Z.00000000016

Skeggs, B. (2011). Imagining personhood differently: Person value and autonomist working-class value practices. *The Sociological Review*, 59(3), 496–513. https://doi.org/10.1111/j.1467-954X.2011.02018.x

Skolbekken, J.-A. (2008). Unlimited medicalization? Risk and the pathologization of normality. In A.R. Petersen and I. Wilkinson (eds), *Health, Risk and Vulnerability* (pp 16–29). Routledge.

Smith, C. and Thompson, P. (1998). Re-evaluating the labour process debate. *Economic and Industrial Democracy*, 19(4), 551–577. https://doi.org/10.1177/0143831X98194002

Smith, R. (1997). *The Norton History of the Human Sciences*. W.W. Norton.

Smith, S.R. and Hamon, R.R. (2012). *Exploring Family Theories*. Oxford University Press.

Social Security Institution of Finland (2022a). *Statistical Database Kelasto*. https://www.kela.fi/web/en/statistical-database-kelasto

Social Security Institution of Finland (2022b). Statistical Database Kelasto. *The Receivers of Rehabilitative Psychotherapy in Finland according to Gender and Age Group in 2011–2021.* https://www.tietotarjotin.fi/tilastodata/2051 231/Tilastotietokanta%20Kelasto

Sommer, M. (2016). *Mental Health among Youth in Sweden: Who is Responsible? What is Being Done?* Nordens välfärdscenter [Nordic Welfare Centre]. http://urn.kb.se/resolve?urn=urn:nbn:se:norden:org:diva-4751

Spitz-Oener, A. (2006). Technical change, job tasks, and rising educational demands: Looking outside the wage structure. *Journal of Labor Economics*, 24(2), 235–270. https://doi.org/10.1086/499972

Standing, G. (2011). *The Precariat: The New Dangerous Class.* Bloomsbury Academic. https://doi.org/10.5040/9781849664554

Standing, G. (2014). *A Precariat Charter: From Denizens to Citizens.* Bloomsbury. https://doi.org/10.5040/9781472510631

Statistics Finland. (2010). *Educational Structure of Population.* Official Statistics of Finland. http://www.stat.fi/til/vkour/2009/vkour_2009_2010-12-03_tie_001_en.html

Stearns, P.N. (1994). *American Cool: Constructing a Twentieth-Century Emotional Style.* New York University Press.

Stearns, P.N. (2010). *Globalization in World History.* Routledge.

Stocks, S.J., McNamee, R., Molen, H.F. van der, Paris, C., Urban, P., Campo, G. et al (2015). Trends in incidence of occupational asthma, contact dermatitis, noise-induced hearing loss, carpal tunnel syndrome and upper limb musculoskeletal disorders in European countries from 2000 to 2012. *Occupational and Environmental Medicine*, 72(4), 294–303. https://doi.org/10.1136/oemed-2014-102534

Strangleman, T. (2007). The nostalgia for permanence at work? The end of work and its commentators. *The Sociological Review*, 55(1), 81–103. https://doi.org/10.1111/j.1467-954X.2007.00683.x

Sullivan, D. (2020). Social psychological theory as history: Outlining the critical-historical approach to theory. *Personality and Social Psychology Review*, 24(1), 78–99. https://doi.org/10.1177/1088868319883174

Sumanen, H., Rahkonen, O., Pietiläinen, O., Lahelma, E., Roos, E. and Lahti, J. (2016). Educational differences in disability retirement among young employees in Helsinki, Finland. *European Journal of Public Health*, 26(2), 318–322. https://doi.org/10.1093/eurpub/ckv226

Sumanen, H., Harkko, J., Lahti, J., Ketonen, E.-L., Pietiläinen, O. and Kouvonen, A. (2020). *Nuorten työntekijöiden työkyky ja työterveyshuollon palvelujen käyttö* [*Young Employees' Working Ability and Usage of Occupational Health Services*] (13; XAMK tutkii). Kaakkois-Suomen ammattikorkeakoulu [South-Eastern Finland University of Applied Sciences]. http://www.theseus.fi/handle/10024/268093

Summers-Effler, E. (2006). Ritual theory. In J.E. Stets and J.H. Turner (eds), *Handbook of the Sociology of Emotions* (pp 135–154). Springer. https://doi.org/10.1007/978-0-387-30715-2_7

Susser, M. (1964). The uses of social science in medicine. *The Lancet*, 284(7357), 425–429. https://doi.org/10.1016/S0140-6736(64)90324-1

Susser, M. (1973). *Causal Thinking in the Health Sciences: Concepts and Strategies of Epidemiology*. Oxford University Press.

Sutela, H. and Lehto, A.-M. (2014). *Työolojen muutokset 1977–2013* [*Changes in Work Conditions in Finland 1977–2013*]. Statistics Finland.

Sutela, H., Pärnänen, A. and Keyriläinen, M. (2019). *Digiajan työelämä: Työolotutkimuksen tuloksia 1977–2018* [*Work Life at the Digitalized Age: Quality of Work Life Survey Results from 1977 to 2018*]. Tilastokeskus.

Suzman, J. (2021). *Work: A Deep History, From the Stone Age to the Age of Robots*. Penguin Press.

Szasz, T.S. (1961). *The Myth of Mental Illness: Foundations of a Theory of Personal Conduct*. Harper & Row.

Tafarodi, R.W. (ed) (2013). *Subjectivity in the Twenty-First Century: Psychological, Sociological, and Political Perspectives*. Cambridge University Press.

Takala, J. (2009). Foreword. In *OSH in Figures: Stress at Work – Facts and Figures*. European Agency for Safety and Health at Work.

Tausig, M. and Fenwick, R. (2011a). Job structures, job stress, and mental health. In M. Tausig and R. Fenwick (eds), *Work and Mental Health in Social Context* (pp 25–49). Springer. https://doi.org/10.1007/978-1-4614-0625-9_2

Tausig, M. and Fenwick, R. (2011b). Work and mental health in social context. In M. Tausig and R. Fenwick (eds), *Work and Mental Health in Social Context* (pp 161–183). Springer. https://doi.org/10.1007/978-1-4614-0625-9_7

Taylor, C. (1992). *The Ethics of Authenticity*. Harvard University Press.

Teo, T. (2023). Subjectivity and work: Critical-theoretical reflections. *Herausgeber/Editor*, 39.

Thoits, P.A. (1985). Self-labeling processes in mental illness: The role of emotional deviance. *The American Journal of Sociology*, 91(2), 221–249. https://doi.org/10.1086/228276

Thoits, P.A. (1989). The sociology of emotions. *Annual Review of Sociology*, 15(1), 317–342. https://doi.org/10.1146/annurev.so.15.080189.001533

Thorsrud, E. (1970). A strategy for research and social change in industry: A report on the Industrial Democracy Project in Norway. *Social Science Information*, 9(5), 64–90. https://doi.org/10.1177/053901847000900504

Tilly, C. (2004). *Social Movements, 1768–2004*. Paradigm Publishers.

Timonen, V. (2003). *Restructuring the Welfare State: Globalization and Social Policy Reform in Finland and Sweden*. Edward Elgar.

Toivanen, M., Viljanen, O. and Turpeinen, M. (2016). Aikamatriiseja asiantuntijatyössä [Time matrices in expert work]. *Työelämän tutkimus* [*Work Life Research*], 14(1), Article 1.

Totton, N. (2006). *The Politics of Psychotherapy: New Perspectives*. Open University Press.

Townsend, P. (1962). The meaning of poverty. *British Journal of Sociology*, 13(3), 210–227. https://doi.org/10.2307/587266

Townsend, P. (1979). *Poverty in the United Kingdom: A Survey of Household Resources and Standards of Living*. Penguin.

Trautmann, S., Rehm, J. and Wittchen, H.-U. (2016). The economic costs of mental disorders: Do our societies react appropriately to the burden of mental disorders? *EMBO Reports*, 17(9), 1245–1249. https://doi.org/10.15252/embr.201642951

Tunestad, H. (2014). *The Therapeutization of Work: The Psychological Toolbox as Rationalization Device during the Third Industrial Revolution in Sweden*. Acta Universitatis Stockholmiensis.

Turkle, S. (1997). *Life on the Screen*. Simon & Schuster.

Turner, N., Barling, J. and Zacharatos, A. (2002). Positive psychology at work. In C.R. Snyder and S.J. Lopez (eds), *Handbook of Positive Psychology*. Oxford University Press, pp 715–728.

Turner, V.W. (1969). *The Ritual Process: Structure and Anti-Structure*. Routledge & Kegan.

Turtiainen, J. and Väänänen, A. (2012). Men of steel? The masculinity of metal industry workers in Finland after World War II. *Journal of Social History*, 46(2), 449–472.

Turtiainen, J., Väänänen, A. and Varje, P. (2018). The pressure of objectives and reality: Social workers' perceptions of their occupational complexities in a trade journal in 1958–1999. *Qualitative Social Work*, 17(6), 849–864. https://doi.org/10.1177/1473325017699453

Turtiainen, J., Anttila, E. and Väänänen, A. (2022). Social work, emotion management and the transformation of the welfare state. *Journal of Social Work*, 22(1), 68–86. https://doi.org/10.1177/1468017320973586

Väänänen, A. and Toivanen, M. (2018). The challenge of tied autonomy for traditional work stress models. *Work and Stress*, 32(1), 1–5. https://doi.org/10.1080/02678373.2017.1415999

Väänänen, A. and Turtiainen, J. (2014). *Suomalainen työntekijyys 1945–2013* [*Finnish Workership from 1945 to 2013*]. Vastapaino.

Väänänen, A., Pahkin, K., Huuhtanen, P., Kivimäki, M., Vahtera, J., Theorell, T. and Kalimo, R. (2005). Are intrinsic motivational factors of work associated with functional incapacity similarly regardless of the country? *Journal of Epidemiology and Community Health*, 59(10), 858–863. https://doi.org/10.1136/jech.2004.030106

Väänänen, A., Anttila, E., Turtiainen, J. and Varje, P. (2012). Formulation of work stress in 1960–2000: Analysis of scientific works from the perspective of historical sociology. *Social Science & Medicine*, 75(5), 784–794. https://doi.org/10.1016/j.socscimed.2012.04.014

Väänänen, A., Murray, M. and Kuokkanen, A. (2014). The growth and the stagnation of work stress: Publication trends and scientific representations 1960–2011. *History of the Human Sciences*, 27(4), 116–138. https://doi.org/10.1177/0952695114525168

Väänänen, A., Koskinen, A. and Toivanen, M. (2016). Korkeakoulutetut asiantuntijat Suomessa [Professionals with high education in Finland]. In M. Toivanen, K. Yli-Kaitala, O. Viljanen, A. Väänänen, M. Turpeinen, M. Janhonen and A. Koskinen (eds), *Aikajärjestys asiantuntijatyössä [(A) Synchrony of Timelines Among Professionals]* (pp 21–30). Finnish Institute of Occupational Health.

Väänänen, A., Turtiainen, J., Kuokkanen, A. and Petersen, A. (2019). From silence to diagnosis: The entry of the mentally problematic employee into medical practice. *Social Theory & Health*, 17(4), 407–426. https://doi.org/10.1057/s41285-019-00101-4

Väänänen, A., Toivanen, M. and Lallukka, T. (2020). Lost in autonomy: Temporal structures and their implications for employees' autonomy and well-being among knowledge workers. *Occupational Health Science*, 4(1–2), 83–101. https://doi.org/10.1007/s41542-020-00058-1

Valkonen, J. and Hänninen, V. (2013). Narratives of masculinity and depression. *Men and Masculinities*, 16(2), 160–180. https://doi.org/10.1177/1097184X12464377

Van Drunen, P. , Hass, E. and Strien, P. (2003). Work and organization. In P. van Drunen and J. Jansz (eds), *A Social History of Psychology* (pp 129–164). Blackwell.

Van Loon, J. (2008). Governmentality and teenage sexual risk behavior. In A.R. Petersen and I. Wilkinson (eds), *Health, Risk and Vulnerability* (pp 48–65). Routledge.

Vannini, P. and Williams, J.P. (2009). *Authenticity in Culture, Self, and Society*. Ashgate.

Varje, P. (2018). *Cracks in the Mirror: The Ideal Worker and the Labor Process in Finnish Working Life After the Second World War*. University of Helsinki.

Varje, P. and Väänänen, A. (2016). Health risks, social relations and class: An analysis of occupational health discourse in Finnish newspaper and women's magazine articles 1961–2008. *Sociology of Health & Illness*, 38(3), 493–510. https://doi.org/10.1111/1467-9566.12376

Varje, P., Anttila, E. and Väänänen, A. (2013a). Emergence of emotional management: Changing manager ideals in Finnish job advertisements from 1949 to 2009. *Management & Organizational History*, 8(3), 245–261. https://doi.org/10.1080/17449359.2013.804416

Varje, P., Turtiainen, J. and Väänänen, A. (2013b). Psychological management: Changing qualities of the ideal manager in Finland 1949–2009. *Journal of Management History*, 19(1), 33–54. https://doi.org/10.1108/17511341311286187

Varje, P., Turtiainen, J., Lehmuskoski, K., Kuokkanen, A. and Väänänen, A. (2021). Mielenterveys työelämän murroskohdissa: Lääketieteellisen intervention muuttuva rooli [Mental health in the turning points of working life: The changing role of the medical intervention]. *Kulttuurintutkimus* [*Cultural Studies*], 38(2–3), Article 2–3.

Vartia, M., Kandolin, I., Toivanen, M., Bergholm, B., Väänänen, A., Pahkin, K., Vesala, H., Haapanen, A. and Viluksela, M. (2012). *Psykososiaaliset tekijät suomalaisessa työyhteisössä* [*Psychosocial Factors in Finnish Work Organizations*]. Ministry of Social Affairs and Health. https://julkaisut.valtioneuvosto.fi/handle/10024/74112

Veenstra, G. (2007). Social space, social class and Bourdieu: Health inequalities in British Columbia, Canada. *Health & Place*, 13(1), 14–31. https://doi.org/10.1016/j.healthplace.2005.09.011

Ventevogel, P. and Faiz, H. (2018). Mental disorder or emotional distress? How psychiatric surveys in Afghanistan ignore the role of gender, culture and context. *Intervention*, 16(3), 207–214. https://doi.org/10.4103/INTV.INTV_60_18

Viola, S. and Moncrieff, J. (2016). Claims for sickness and disability benefits owing to mental disorders in the UK: Trends from 1995 to 2014. *BJPsych Open*, 2(1), 18–24. https://doi.org/10.1192/bjpo.bp.115.002246

Virkki, T. (2008). The art of pacifying an aggressive client: 'Feminine' skills and preventing violence in caring work. *Gender, Work, and Organization*, 15(1), 72–87. https://doi.org/10.1111/j.1468-0432.2007.00365.x

Virokannas, E., Liuski, S. and Kuronen, M. (2020). The contested concept of vulnerability: A literature review. *European Journal of Social Work*, 23(2), 327–339. https://doi.org/10.1080/13691457.2018.1508001

Voloshinov, V.N. (1986). *Marxism and the Philosophy of Language*. Harvard University Press.

Vosko, L.F. (2009). *Managing the Margins: Gender, Citizenship, and the International Regulation of Precarious Employment*. Oxford University Press.

Voutilainen, R. (2005). Comparing alternative structures of financial alliances. *The Geneva Papers on Risk and Insurance. Issues and Practice*, 30(2), 327–342.

Vygotsky, L.S. (1962). *Thought and Language*. MIT Press.

Wagner, G. (2017). Exhaustion and euphoria: Self-medication with amphetamines. In S. Neckel, A.K. Schaffner, and G. Wagner (eds), *Burnout, Fatigue, Exhaustion: An Interdisciplinary Perspective on a Modern Affliction* (pp 195–216). Springer.

Wainwright, D. and Calnan, M. (2002). *Work Stress: The Making of a Modern Epidemic*. Open University Press.

Wainwright, D. and Calnan, M. (2011). The fall of work stress and the rise of wellbeing. In S. Vickerstaff, C. Phillipson and R. Wilkie (eds), *Work, Health and Wellbeing: The Challenges of Managing Health at Work* (pp 161–186). Policy Press.

Wajcman, J. and Rose, E. (2011). Constant connectivity: Rethinking interruptions at work. *Organization Studies*, 32(7), 941–961. https://doi.org/10.1177/0170840611410829

Ward, J. and McMurray, R. (2015). *The Dark Side of Emotional Labour*. Routledge.

Warr, P.G. (1987). *Work, Unemployment, and Mental Health*. Clarendon Press.

Warr, P.G. (2007). Some historical developments in I-O psychology outside the United States. In L. Koppes (ed), *Historical Perspectives in Industrial and Organizational Psychology* (pp 81–107). Psychology Press.

Weber, M. (1978). *Economy and Society: An Outline of Interpretive Sociology*. University of California Press.

Webster, J. (Director). (2022). *The Happy Worker*. Yellow Film & TV.

Weckroth, K. (2020). *Kaiken järjen mukaan* [*Viewed Rationally*]. BoB- Books on Demand.

Weiskopf, R. and Munro, I. (2012). Management of human capital: Discipline, security and controlled circulation in HRM. *Organization*, 19(6), 685–702. https://doi.org/10.1177/1350508411416536

West, C. and Zimmerman, D.H. (1987). Doing gender. *Gender & Society*, 1(2), 125–151. https://doi.org/10.1177/0891243287001002002

Wettergren, Å. and Sieben, B. (2010). *Emotionalizing Organizations and Organizing Emotions*. Palgrave Macmillan.

WHO (2002). *Gender and Mental Health*. WHO. https://apps.who.int/iris/handle/10665/68884

WHO (2014). *Global Health Estimates 2014 Summary Tables: YLD by Cause, Age and Sex, Region, 2000–2012*. WHO.

WHO (2017). *Depression and Other Common Mental Disorders* (WHO/MSD/MER/2017.2; Global Health Estimates). WHO. https://apps.who.int/iris/handle/10665/254610

Whyte, W.H. (1956). *The Organization Man*. Touchstone.

Wilkinson, I. (2009). *Risk, Vulnerability and Everyday Life*. Routledge.

Wilkinson, I. (2017). Social agony and agonising social constructions. In S. Neckel, A.K. Schaffner and G. Wagner (eds), *Burnout, Fatigue, Exhaustion: An Interdisciplinary Perspective on a Modern Affliction* (pp 259–283). Springer.

Wilkinson, I. and Väänänen, A. (2021). The informalization of doctor–patient relations in a Finnish setting: New social figurations and emergent possibilities. *Sociology of Health & Illness*, 43(9), 1965–1980. https://doi.org/10.1111/1467-9566.13375

Wilkinson, R.G. (2000). Inequality and the social environment: A reply to Lynch et al. *Journal of Epidemiology & Community Health*, 54(6), 411–413. https://doi.org/10.1136/jech.54.6.411

Williams, D.R. (2003). The health of men: Structured inequalities and opportunities. *American Journal of Public Health*, 93(5), 724–731. https://doi.org/10.2105/AJPH.93.5.724

Williams, R. (1961). *The Long Revolution*. Chatto & Windus.

Williams, R. (1980). *Problems in Materialism and Culture: Selected Essays*. Verso.

Williams, S.J., Gabe, J. and Davis, P. (2008). The sociology of pharmaceuticals: Progress and prospects. *Sociology of Health & Illness*, 30(6), 813–824. https://doi.org/10.1111/j.1467-9566.2008.01123.x

Wisner, B. and Luce, H.R. (1993). Disaster vulnerability: Scale, power and daily life. *GeoJournal*, 30(2), 127–140. https://doi.org/10.1007/BF00808129

Wittchen, H.-U. and Jacobi, F. (2005). Size and burden of mental disorders in Europe: A critical review and appraisal of 27 studies. *European Neuropsychopharmacology*, 15(4), 357–376. https://doi.org/10.1016/j.euroneuro.2005.04.012

Witz, A., Warhurst, C. and Nickson, D. (2003). The labour of aesthetics and the aesthetics of organization. *Organization*, 10(1), 33–54. https://doi.org/10.1177/1350508403010001375

Womack, J.P., Jones, D.T. and Roos, D. (1990). *The Machine that Changed the World: The Story of Lean Production – Toyota's Secret Weapon in the Global Car Wars That Is Revolutionizing World Industry*. Free Press.

Wouters, C. (1986). Formalization and informalization: Changing tension balances in civilizing processes. *Theory, Culture & Society*, 3(2), 1–18. https://doi.org/10.1177/0263276486003002002

Wouters, C. (1992). On status competition and emotion management: The study of emotions as a new field. *Theory, Culture & Society*, 9(1), 229–252. https://doi.org/10.1177/026327692009001012

Wouters, C. (2007). *Informalization: Manners and Emotions Since 1890*. SAGE.

Wouters, C. (2011). How civilizing processes continued: Towards an informalization of manners and a third nature personality. *The Sociological Review*, 59(s1), 140–159. https://doi.org/10.1111/j.1467-954X.2011.01982.x

Ybema, S.B., Keenoy, T., Oswick, C., Beverungen, A., Ellis, N. and Sabelis, I.H.J. (2009). Articulating identities. *Human Relations*, 62(3), 299–322. https://doi.org/10.1177/0018726708101904

Young, A. (1980). The discourse on stress and the reproduction of conventional knowledge. *Social Science & Medicine*, 14(3), 133–146. https://doi.org/10.1016/0160-7987(80)90003-4

Zembylas, M. (2006). Challenges and possibilities in a postmodern culture of emotions in education. *Interchange*, 37(3), 251–275. https://doi.org/10.1007/s10780-006-9003-y

Ziehe, T. (1991). *Uusi nuoriso: Epätavanomaisen oppimisen puolustus* [*The New Youth: A Defence of Unconventional Learning*]. Vastapaino.

Żołnierczyk-Zreda, D., Bedyńska, S. and Warszewska-Makuch, M. (2012). Work time control and mental health of workers working long hours: The role of gender and age. *International Journal of Occupational Safety and Ergonomics*, 18(3), 311–320. https://doi.org/10.1080/10803 548.2012.11076947

Zubin, J. and Spring, B. (1977). Vulnerability: A new view of schizophrenia. *Journal of Abnormal Psychology*, 86(2), 103–126.

Index

Printed and bound by CPI Group (UK) Ltd, Croydon, CR0 4YY

16/04/2025

14658340-0004